CW00551657

Susan Curtis has worked with natural medicines since 1979. She originally trained as a homœopath, and has since studied and used other forms of natural healing including herbs and essential oils. Susan practices homœopathy professionally at a clinic of natural medicine in London. She is a co-author of *Neal's Yard Natural Remedies* and *Natural Healing for Women* and author of *Homœopathic Alternatives to Immunisation*. Susan has two children and lives in Kent.

Surviving
with
Natural
Remedies

Susan Curtis RSHom

Winter Press
16 Stambourne Way
West Wickham
Kent BR4 9NF
e-mail: winterpress@hotmail.com

First published by Winter Press in 2003

© Susan Curtis 2003

ISBN 1 874581 32 0

Printed by Biddles of Guildford, Surrey

ACKNOWLEDGMENTS

With grateful thanks for their valuable contributions to Janice Micallef, Romy Fraser, Peter Chappell, Nick Churchill, Wendy Davies and Julian Barker. Also to my husband, Colin Winter, for his help and support.

CONTENTS

INTRODUCTION

This book was written out of the thought, "what happens when there are no reliable emergency services or effective medical help". There are a number of reasons why that situation may arise. In developing countries, there may simply not be the resources available. Even in more affluent countries a serious disaster may swamp the emergency services, at least for a time. Or people may want to supplement what is offered by the authorities with complementary remedies, such as herbs or homœopathy. There are also those who choose to live in a more self-reliant way, and prefer to avoid orthodox medicine and its links with pharmaceutical corporations.

The book was started before the terrorist attacks of September 11th 2001 and the events that followed, but all of that has certainly brought home the fact that none of us are immune to the times we live in.

This is in no way meant to be a book that further contributes to the fear that is prevalent, rather it is a practical guide for those people that choose not to feel helpless however dire the situation. There are always those people that find the strength to make the most of their own situation and to help others, even in extreme circumstances.

You may find this book helpful to have "just in case" you need it for yourself and your family, although I hope it will be most useful to those people actually working in disaster situations, for example, relief workers open to using natural remedies, teachers and anyone whom people come to for help. It will also be of use to qualified practitioners who may not have much experience in treating during disaster situations, but find they need to adapt their skills to meet more extreme needs when they arise.

In many poor parts of the world, medical and pharmaceutical resources are extremely limited for most of the population because they are too expensive or simply not available. One of the great advantages of natural remedies is that they are relatively inexpensive (herbs and homœopathy) and ecologically sustainable (especially homœopathy).

One of the beauties of herbal medicine is that the raw materials may be found in virtually every part of the world. Medicinal herbs can be found in urban, suburban and rural environments, in hot and cool countries. When researching this book, I interviewed someone who was employed by the Royal Marines during the conflict

1

in former Yugoslavia, to teach his colleagues about the use of such herbs as calendula and yarrow that were growing in the area. The SAS Handbook has a section on plants for wild food and medicine in survival situations.

When looking at the alternatives to pharmaceuticals, one has to ask, "how effective are natural remedies", and, "how far can we rely on them"? Few reliable trials have been carried out to determine exact efficacy rates for natural remedies. There are an increasing number of trials showing the efficacy of herbs, notably in Germany, but there are very few satisfactory trials on homœopathy. There have been some studies done using homœopathic prophylaxis for preventing contagious diseases, eg. an eminent homœopath, Dorothy Shepherd, states that the homœopathic remedy Pertussin was given daily for 2 weeks to 364 cases after contact with whooping cough and not one child contracted the disease. There are also several accounts in current farming journals of homœopathic vets getting excellent results by giving farm animals homœopathic nosodes to prevent common farm diseases.

As always with alternative medicine there is a lot more anecdotal evidence for cures than there are trial results. For example, thousands of children have been treated with homœopathy in Russia since the Chernobyl disaster and several homœopaths have written of their experiences in homœopathic journals. Similarly, a number of charities, including Frontline Homeopathy, have trained health care workers in using homœopathy to treat post-traumatic stress disorder following disasters, and this has well-reported successes.

The US Government has considered the use of homœopathy when discussing medical care for the victims of biological warfare. Dr Wayne Jonas MD, former director of the Office of Alternative Medicine at the National Institute of Health, is among those who have testified before a House Government Reform Committee set up to coordinate medical care during attacks with biological weapons. He said they should consider the use of homœopathic medicines for both viral and bacterial illnesses associated with bio-terror. The same committee also considered the use of homœopathy for anthrax following the anthrax attacks of 2001. Sales of the homœopathic remedy Anthracinum multiplied after September 2001, and Joyce Frye DO, MBA, President-Elect, American Institute of Homœopathy described case histories for the homœopathic treatment of anthrax in humans (see Footnote 1).

There is a strong bibliographic tradition of the use of herbs and homœopathic remedies for treating conditions that were prevalent in the past and particularly from the 19th and early 20th centuries. First aid conditions are well covered and also some of the epidemic illnesses that it is feared may reemerge again, such as smallpox and cholera. In other instances, such as poisoning with chemicals, there is little direct experience to draw on but the principles for the appropriate approach to take are similar to previously encountered and well-recorded situations.

It may be that you use the natural remedies suggested in this book in conjunction with orthodox treatments. That indeed could be the best option in certain situations. If accident and emergency treatment is available, for example after a bomb blast, then the best results will be obtained by receiving attention from the paramedics and taking Arnica and using other natural remedies as appropriate.

A study from Germany on pig herds, particularly susceptible to infections due to their crowded growing conditions, showed that a homœopathic combination remedy was just as effective as prophylactic doses of antibiotic. Full doses of antibiotic were more effective, but carry the risk of greater side effects and bacterial immunity developing (see Footnote 2). This could indicate that in low risk categories the sensible approach would be to use homœopathic prophylaxis, but in high risk categories, eg. following confirmed contact, high doses of antibiotics may be advisable if available. After the disease has been treated, then natural remedies may again be used to relieve the side effects of high dose medication.

The point is that survival is all about adaptability, and there is a wealth of information about natural remedies that can be useful to us for modern day survival. There are conditions where natural remedies may be the only available form of treatment in an extreme situation, or they may be used alongside conventional medical treatment to enhance its effects. I have been fortunate to have worked with natural medicine for more than 20 years, and seen first hand the amazing effectiveness of natural treatment of very serious conditions both in the UK and in places such as India and North Africa. Natural medicine can become part of your everyday life but also an incredible resource to improve health, welfare and survival in extreme situations.

Footnotes
1. "Germ Warfare: Can Homeopathy Protect", CAM Magazine, January 2002, Issue 6.
2. Schutt, A., "Homeopathy versus Antibiotics in Metaphylaxis of Infectious Diseases", Alternative Therapies, 1999, 5:64-68.

PART I

IF THE WORST SHOULD HAPPEN

SURVIVAL

In this part we will deal with some of those dire emergencies that can affect large groups of people. It is a sad fact that in recent decades the following events have all been experienced by huge numbers of people: natural disasters including earthquakes, hurricanes and floods; man made disasters including chemical leaks, explosions, hijackings; war with conventional weapons and biological and chemical warfare. Radiation fallout from both bombs and power plant leaks have also affected millions.

Obviously in all these situations, the initial response is pure survival. Getting away from the epicentre of the crisis and immediate first-aid are the prime factors. Survival will be related to timing, position, skill and will power.

The next stage is to effectively deal with injuries and shock. There may or may not be emergency services to assist. Following that, making the most of the resources available will be necessary to find water, food and shelter, and to treat psychological trauma and physical injuries. Prevention of infection and taking steps to establish adequate sanitation thus preventing the outbreak of contagious diseases, will be of key importance.

The use of natural remedies can be supremely helpful in such conditions. Some specific situations are discussed in this chapter; you should also refer to the section in the appendices on first-aid and acute illnesses. Obviously you will have to use what you have available, this is why this book tries to make the most use out of a limited number of some of the more common remedies. If an aid-worker is going into an area they can take supplies with them. It is not within the scope of this book to give comprehensive first-aid treatments for every situation (although see Explosions and Gunshot, etc. below). For more detailed advice see the remarkable book, "Where There Is No Doctor", by David Werner.

NATURAL DISASTERS

Floods, hurricanes, earthquakes and wars can kill and injure people and also cause people to lose their homes and livelihood. The past few decades have seen many situations where whole communities have had to abandon their homes and seek refuge elsewhere.

Just one example was Hurricane Mitch, which struck in November 1998 and devastated Honduras and Nicaragua. Peter Chappell, then Director of Frontline Homœopathy, visited the region immediately afterwards to deliver remedies and train local health care workers. He reported, "People watched the land they owned, their houses, their crops and even their families being washed away in the storms...There was no food, wells were contaminated and blocked, livestock were killed or missing. Crops which were just about to be harvested had been totally destroyed."

POST-TRAUMATIC STRESS

In addition to the physical injuries that need treatment, the potential for psychological damage is immense. Following the trauma of a terrifying ordeal many have to face the loss of family members. Again in the words of Peter Chappell following Hurricane Mitch, "Everyone had suffered. There were various stages of shock, denial, insecurity. The people in the shelters were suffering from the psychological stress of being confined in a crowded place on top of major trauma."

The most useful homœopathic remedies in such situations are:

Aconite: Shock and panic. The idea, "I will die any minute."

Arsenicum alb: Profound insecurity, fear. Follows loss of possessions.

Ignatia: Grief with denial and sighing. Hysteria.

Natrum mur: Grief and denial of it. Bottled up.

Opium: Confusion. Panic.

Phosphoric acid: Worn out and run down from grief. No feelings left.

Staphysagria: Victims, passed by. Smile sweetly.

Stramonium: Terror of being again in a very dangerous situation. Dread of darkness – must have the light on.

For more details see the Remedy section. Anyone with a working knowledge of just these homœopathic remedies (especially in conjunction with the major first-aid remedies) could do an enormous amount to relieve the symptoms of acute stress and trauma following a major natural disaster.

EXPLOSIONS AND GUNSHOT, ETC

The twentieth century saw millions of people killed and injured by terrorism and warfare. War causes devastation physically, psychologically and culturally. The remedies listed above under Post-Traumatic Stress, can be used to treat some of the psychological effects of being caught up in a war or after experiencing the trauma of an explosion or shooting.

To treat the physical effects see First Aid, page 94. A special consideration is that any deep bullet, shrapnel or knife wound runs a high risk of dangerous infection. The following points are general to all severe injuries, obviously the chances of survival will be massively increased if it is possible for the patient to receive experienced medical treatment very quickly.

To Control Bleeding

- Raise the injured part
- With a clean cloth, piece of clothing, or your hand if nothing else is available, press directly on the wound. Keep pressing until the bleeding stops. This may take up to 20 minutes. This type of direct pressure combined with raising the injured part will nearly always stop the bleeding even if part of the body has been cut off.
- If there is bleeding from many areas, or injury is severe, raise the feet and lower the head to help prevent shock.
- Give homœopathic Arnica to help reduce haemorrhage and prevent shock. If bleeding is/has been profuse give homœopathic China.

To Prevent Infection

- Wash wounds well with boiled water and soap. Remove all pieces of dirt, blood clots or badly damaged flesh. Use tweezers (boil in water for 20 minutes to sterilise first) if necessary.
- Allow the wound to dry in the air, only use a dressing if there is risk of further dust or dirt entering the wound. Never use a dressing that is wet or dirty.
- Give homœopathic Arnica to promote healing and help prevent infection.
- If the wound is deep use what medicines you have available to prevent infection: antibiotics, antimicrobial herbs, homœopathic remedies for infection, etc., (see First Aid, page 94).
- Do not use alcohol or any undiluted tinctures directly on a wound. Doing so damages the flesh and delays healing.
- Do not attempt to close a large wound with stitches or 'butterfly' plasters (infection may start underneath).
- The danger of tetanus is very great in deep wounds. Consider vaccination or homœopathic prophylaxis (Ledum).

Injuries to Specific Parts of the Body

LIMBS:

- Control heavy bleeding using pressure (described above).
- Wash the wound with boiled water and soap. Do not poke anything into the hole, eg. trying to remove a bullet.

- Take remedies to prevent infection.
- If a bullet has hit the leg try not to walk on it. If the bullet has hit the bone any weight on the leg may worsen a break. If the bone has been broken the leg will need a splint for several weeks.
- Keep the affected limb in a raised postion. If a leg, lie or sit with the leg raised on cusions, etc. An arm should be supported with a sling.
- Give homœopathic Arnica. If the pain is very severe or nerves damaged give homœopathic Hypericum.

HEAD:
- Cover the wound with a clean dressing.
- Place the person so they are in the 'half sitting' postion, ie lying down with cusions or clothes propping up their head and shoulders.
- Give homœopathic Arnica and Natrum sulph. Give further remedies to prevent infection.
- Seek urgent medical help.

CHEST:
- Allow the patient to rest in the most comfortable position.
- If the wound has reached the lungs and air is being sucked through when the person breathes, cover the hole immediately. Spread Vaseline or vegetable fat on a clean pad, place it over the hole and keep it in place by wrapping a bandage around the chest.
- Give homœopathic Arnica and further remedies to prevent infection.
- Seek medical help.

ABDOMEN:
- Cover the wound with a clean dressing.
- If the guts are partly outside the wound do not try to push them back in. Cover them with a clean cloth soaked in lightly salted, cool boiled water. Keep the cloth wet.
- Lay the person down with their feet higher than their head to prevent shock.
- Give no food or drink by mouth. If it will take more than two days to get medical attention give only small sips of water.
- Give homœopathic Arnica and further remedies to prevent infection.
- Seek urgent medical help. Surgery will most likely be necessary.

CHEMICAL DISASTERS

This is difficult to write about, because whilst such poisonings happen, there is little evidence available of the use of natural remedies to treat the immediate symptoms. There is more information available about the homœopathic treatment of the long term side-effects of exposure to toxic substances. Examples of recent occurences of this kind of disaster include factory chemical leaks, the largest of which has been Bhopal in India. Accidental chemical contamination of the drinking water supply, the best known example of which happened in Camelford, Cornwall; and exposure to excessive chlorine in public swimming pools, of which there were two reported major incidents in the UK in 1999 alone.

There is also the horrific use of chemical and biological weapons during warfare and terrorist attacks. Following the terrorist attacks of September 11th in the USA tens of people contracted anthrax from spores sent in the post. These incidents have created a widespread awareness and fear of the possibility of further attacks such as the dissemination of smallpox and contamination of reservoirs.

CHEMICAL POISONINGS

The obvious thing should be stated; remove yourself from the source of contamination as rapidly as possible. By their nature most chemicals are dose dependent, so the greater and more prolonged the dose, the worse the damage that will be done.

If the contamination is airborne, go/stay indoors and tape up windows and air vents for as long as possible. If there is smoke or visible particles then wet a cloth (eg. tea towel), wring it out and tie it round your mouth and nose so that you breath through the damp cloth. This can act as a filter for larger molecules.

Ensure that nothing is put in the mouth that may have been exposed to the contaminant eg. fingers, pencils. Make sure that young children do not put a comforter or toy that may have been exposed in their mouth.

If poisonous substances have been ingested it is usually beneficial to drink lots of clean water to flush them through. If the substance is known to be very alkaline, eg. caustic soda, then it is more beneficial to drink milk to help neutralise it.

If the source is known to be petrochemical or corrosive, do not attempt to induce vomiting. Also do not attempt to induce vomiting if the victim is unconscious.

If the skin has been affected it is usually best, if possible, to shower or bathe the area in copious amounts of cool water.

Herbal Remedies
(For further details look the herbs up in the Remedy section)
Internal poisoning: drink infusions of Chamomile, Liquorice or
Slippery Elm.
External irritation: apply a cold poultice of Comfrey, Plantain,
Marshmallow or Slippery Elm.
Consider also Echinacea internally and externally to prevent
infection.

Homœopathic Remedies
Following immediate exposure and to alleviate shock and panic
give one of the following:
Aconite: Terror, panic, feeling will die any minute.
Arnica: Shock, trauma. Helps kickstart healing process.
Arsenicum alb: Fear. Breathing difficulties following chemical
exposure.
In cases of obvious poisoning use the poison in potency (by obtain-
ing from a homœopathic pharmacy or making yourself).

BIOLOGICAL DISASTERS
Biological weapons are one of the most frightening prospects of
modern warfare. Nations at war, terrorist groups and even deter-
mined individuals can and have cultivated disease organisms such
as smallpox and anthrax. Fortunately it has proved much harder
to widely disseminate the diseases, than it has to manufacture
them. Anthrax spores, sent in the post in the USA during 2001,
apparently affected only those journalists and postal workers that
directly handled them. To date the rumours and fears of using
crop sprayers, air conditioning units and aerosols to spread contagious diseases have proved unfounded.

ANTHRAX
Anthrax is an infectious disease passed among animals. Humans
can contract the disease by contact with infected animals or animal
parts, eg. bones, hides and wool. The disease is caused by the
anthrax bacillus, Bacillus anthracis. 'Natural' outbreaks occur most
commonly in farming areas of Australia, Russia and South America.
Once in the environment, highly resistant spores may persist for
centuries.
   In terms of symptoms, there are two types of anthrax, external
and internal. The external type can occur by infection through
cracks and cuts in the skin; a 'boil' appears on the area, and the
inflammation area spreads until a small area of pus appears in the

middle that bursts to produce a black scab about half an inch in diameter. If unchecked, this malignant pustule may progress to septicaemia. In the internal type, caused by breathing in the spores of the bacillus, or eating infected flesh, acute pneumonia or gastroenteritis develops. Whatever the point of entry, anthrax symptoms are pronounced by their putridity and malignancy, leading to toxaemia and septicaemia in the victim.

The incubation period is between two days and two weeks, depending on the magnitude of exposure. The fatality rates are estimated as 20% for external anthrax and greater than 80% for internal anthrax.

Orthodox treatment is with antibiotics, which have been moderately effective in the treatment of external anthrax providing the disease is diagnosed early and treatment is prolonged. Orthodox treatment of anthrax of the lungs has not been successful, as demonstrated by the fatalities from the postal anthrax attacks in the USA in 2001. Vaccines appear to offer reasonable protection in small exposures providing the vaccination is given prior to exposure, and must be considered for individuals at high risk. The spores of the bacillus may lie latent in the lungs, to germinate at a later time.

Natural remedies can be used to support orthodox treatment, or may be tried if orthodox treatment is not available or decided against. The homœopathic literature has many examples of the successful treatment of both internal and external anthrax, mainly from the early 20th century when orthodox alternatives were not available. (Allen, H.C., Materia Medica of the Nosodes, Jain, 1910; Clarke, J.H., Dictionary of Materia Medica, Health Science Press, 1900). More recently in a Reuters communication, Dr B. Gangapadhyay, former head of the Orissa Medical College of Homeopathy and Research, has reported the successful use of Anthracinum nosode as a preventative measure in humans for anthrax.

Treatment of Anthrax

Anecdotal evidence suggests that Echinacea was used in the past with success in the USA in the treatment of anthrax. Bartram quotes a pioneer herbalist successfully prescribing Echinacea liquid extract: 1 teaspoonful every 4 hours day and night. (Bartram, T., Encyclopedia of Herbal Medicine, Grace, 1995)

HOMŒOPATHIC REMEDIES MOST LIKELY TO BE INDICATED ARE:

Anthracinum, Arsenicum alb, Secale

These should be looked up in the Remedy section.

Prevention
The homœopathic nosode, Anthracinum, should be given in the
30th potency twice a week for 6 weeks following suspected exposure or as an adjunct to other remedies during treatment.

PLAGUE
The Black Death casts a long shadow throughout history; but in
modern times, better hygiene, increased sanitation and treatment
with antibiotics have kept any isolated incidents contained. It
appears the only risk of an epidemic occurring again comes from
deliberate contamination, as from a war or terrorist situation, or
following the collapse of medical and waste disposal services provided by governments.

Plague is caused by infection with the micro-organism Yersinia
pestis. This normally affects rats and other rodents, but the rat
flea, which harbours Yersinia pestis can infect humans, either by
handling live or dead animals, or if the flea seeks a new host and
is unable to find a rodent. Transmission may also occur by droplet
spread from a human sufferer; this causes pneumonic plague,
which is highly contagious.

Plague is currently endemic in South America, India, China, and
parts of Africa, although outbreaks are contained.

The incubation period for plague is two to seven days, and then
the symptoms of severe headache, shivering, dizziness, fever, delirium and rapid pulse develop. An intense facial expression and
confused speech are characteristic. In the classic form of plague,
called bubonic plague, glands of the body enlarge and may sup-
purate (called buboes), and haemorrhagic spots break out on the
skin. Pneumonia may occur as a complication of bubonic plague,
or as a primary pneumonic plague. In primary septicaemic plague
the infection spreads so rapidly in the blood, that the patient usually dies within three days, before any buboes develop.

The mortality rate in cases of untreated plague is 65-95%.
Antibiotics have proved to be effective in many cases providing
they are started early enough. Natural remedies may be given
alongside antibiotics, or if the latter are not available.

Treatment and Prevention of Plague
The best known plant remedy for preventing plague is to eat raw
garlic. During the Black Death there is anecdotal evidence that
those households which ate raw Garlic every day escaped infection. Whilst this may seem archaic, Garlic is a very effective
antimicrobial and this may be taken in conjunction with other
measures.

American herbalists record the use of Echinacea and Wild Indigo internally in the treatment of plague. Externally, Bartram recommends a poultice of Slippery Elm, Marshmallow or Plantain to promote suppuration in bubonic plague. Lancing of buboes is not recommended, as it tends to spread the infection.

Homœopathic remedies that are most likely to be indicated in plague include: Arsenicum album, Crotalus horridus, Ignatia, Lachesis, Phosphorus, Pyrogen, Tarentula cubensis

Homœopathic Prevention
Take the nosode Yersinia pestis 30th potency twice a week during an epidemic.

SMALLPOX
Smallpox is an acute infectious fever caused by the Variola virus. Infection is spread by contact or inhalation of the virus found in the fluid of the pocks. The incubation period is 10-14 days.

The onset of symptoms is usually sudden, with a headache, pronounced backache, vomiting and a high temperature. Often there is a 'prodromal' reddish rash before the true rash appears on the third day. When the true rash appears the temperature usually falls back to normal, and the rash appears as spots which turn into blisters and then pustules. During the pustular stage (during the second week) the temperature rises again and the pustules burst, usually after about two weeks, forming crusts. The crusts leave indented scars.

The rash first appears on the extremities (legs, arms and scalp), and then slowly moves on to the body (this is the opposite of the milder chickenpox that starts on the trunk and moves out to the extremities).

When the pustules remain more or less separated from each other, the outlook for the patient is good. Where the pustules join together, and may form abscesses, the patient will feel very unwell with a high fever and the prognosis is grave. In some cases there is bleeding into the pustules and haemorrhages from the mucous membranes, and this type of haemorrhagic smallpox is the most fatal type. The death rate from smallpox varies from about 0.2% to 15% depending on the strain.

Smallpox has been eradicated since the late 1970s, probably partly through vaccination programs and partly through more effective isolation nursing. Vaccination is undertaken by inoculating the skin with fluid from a vesicle containing the Vaccinia (cowpox) virus taken from calves. Because there have been no outbreaks of smallpox in recent years, vaccination is no longer carried out routinely. It has been postulated that smallpox is potentially a disease that may be spread by terrorists, although there is to date no evidence of that.

There is no specific orthodox treatment for smallpox, although efforts are concentrated at preventing secondary infection from the pustules. Isolation of patients and nursing staff for 6 weeks or until all scabs have healed is essential to prevent the spread of this highly infectious disease.

Vaccination does appear to be effective against smallpox although those with active skin disease, eg. infantile eczema cannot be vaccinated since they may develop a generalised vaccinia which could be fatal. Also vaccination should not be undertaken during pregnancy owing to the danger of damage to the foetus.

Homœopathy has a good record in the prevention of smallpox. For example, Dr Charles Eaton reported on his experiences to the American Institute of Homœopathy in 1907: he stated that of the 2,806 people protected by the homœopathic remedy, 547 were definitely exposed to smallpox, but only 14 were subsequently affected; a 97% effectiveness rate. (Gilruth, C., "The Heroic Uses of Homeopathy in Epidemics", The Homeopath, April 2002, No 85)

Homœopathic Remedies
Ant tart - Earlier stages

Crotalus horridus - Malignant/haemorrhagic

Merc sol - Pustular stage

Homœopathic Prevention: Variolinum 30

Take twice a week following exposure or suspected exposure. Also take to relieve symptoms of active smallpox.

RADIATION

Ever since the discovery of X-rays in the late 1890s, we have been exposed to steadily increasing doses of high energy radiation. As well as being used in medicine, these radiations have been finding progressively wider uses in industry, airports, agriculture, power stations and weapons. Unfortunately, the great energy that makes them so useful also makes them a great hazard to living organisms.

The large and elaborately structured molecules of the living cell appear to be especially sensitive to damage by radiation. Radiation particles carry an electrical charge that disturb the body's molecular and atomic electrons in their orbits, causing ionization and a resultant series of destructive biochemical reactions. Cell membranes can be ruptured, electrical potentials disturbed, structural proteins such as collagen damaged and DNA can be disrupted. The result is that damage may find its expression in gross harm and death to the exposed organism, or it may be transmitted as an hereditary defect to the offspring.

Those tissues that reproduce most rapidly are more open to the immediate symptoms of radiation. This includes red and white blood cells (thereby involving the spleen and bone marrow), the cells of the intestinal linings, and those in the basal layers of the skin.

Children and developing embryos are particularly at risk, because their active growth will immediately proliferate any damage that is done to their cells. Mutations are also highly likely in the reproductive germ cells, and any genetic disruption at this stage of development will result in abnormalities to some degree in future offspring. In adults the effects can be immediate, or may not show up for as much as twenty or thirty years. The exposure to low levels of radiation in particular is known to cause cancers many years in the future.

RADIATION SICKNESS

When a single heavy dose of radiation is received - as it was at Hiroshima and Nagasaki during WWII - then symptoms of radiation sickness will precede other signs of cellular damage. The victims can be divided into three groups according to the dose received. The following chart summarises the course of sickness for those three groups.

One of the remarkable things about radiation sickness is that, apart from attacks of severe vomiting and lethargy that occur within an hour or so after irradiation, the victim has no immediate indication that he has received a fatal or near fatal dose. This very early nausea is a physiological response to the radiation and its duration is usually only two or three days. The radiation affects the neuro-muscular system of the intestine, which then appears to return to normal for a period of time.

If a dose in excess of 800 rems has been received, death is almost certain, and from four to five days after exposure the patient will become obviously very ill. His temperature will rise and he loses weight very quickly. The linings of the stomach and intestines have become so severely damaged that food can no longer be absorbed. Within two weeks or a month at most, death occurs.

Symptoms of Radiation Sickness
From observations made in Japan

Time after exposure	800 rems (Lethal dose)	700 rems (medium lethal dose)	200 rems (moderate dose)
First week	Nausea and vomiting after 2 hours		No definite symptoms
	No definite symptoms	No definite symptoms	
	Diarrhoea, vomiting, inflammation of the throat		
Second week	Fever, rapid emaciation leading to death (100%)		
Third week		Loss of hair. Loss of appetite. General malaise. Fever and pallor leading to rapid emaciation and death for 50% of population	Loss of hair. Loss of appetite. Pallor and diarrhoea. Recovery begins (no deaths in the absence of complications)

The so called critical dose in a single irradiation is about 100 rems, and below this no immediate symptoms such as vomiting or general lethargy are observed.

Symptoms of radiation sickness may also occur following repeated irradiation with lower intensities. This occurs, for example, following medical radiation therapy.

REMEDIES FOR RADIATION EXPOSURE

There is a great deal that can be done using natural remedies to treat someone who has received less than a fatal dose of radiation. Our information is based on recovery rates following the atomic bombs in Hiroshima and Nagasaki, the treatment of the side-effects of medical radiation therapy and the results of animal testing (which must obviously be used with caution). Since the Chernobyl nuclear reactor meltdown in 1986, there has also been much good work done with survivors and especially the children of the area, by both homœopaths and nutritionists. However, it should also be stated that whilst the remedies can help to reduce or modify the effects of radiation, nothing can totally undo those effects, and this is truly a case where prevention has to be better than cure.

Since the Gulf War in 1991, cancer, leukaemia and birth malformations in southern Iraq have risen by 66%. According to "Environmental and Health News", Kuwait and Saudi Arabia are experiencing similar problems in areas used by US soldiers for training, as are Gulf War veterans and their children in the UK and US. The most likely cause of all this is the depleted uranium (DU) used by the UK and US forces to make their deadly weapons even more lethal. Similar problems are projected in Serbia and Kosovo following the UN bombings there during 1999.

Nutritional Supplements

ANTIOXIDANTS:
One of the ionizing effects of radiation is to release free radicals and free electrons that cause a cascade of damage within the cells. Therefore it is the antioxidants, which absorb these molecules and electrons, that are of most help. The key antioxidant vitamins are vitamin C (1-3g daily) and vitamin E (400-800iu). Other supplements of major importance in protecting against radiation damage are selenium, pantothenic acid, calcium and magnesium.

IODINE:
Radioactive iodine is one of the cocktail of radioactive components that was released by Chernobyl. Because the thyroid gland

in the neck will store iodine for use when required (for up to 4 months), it is considered beneficial to take iodine supplements (500-800mcg daily) to top up the available storage space before the radioactive variety comes along in the food chain.

Plants and Foods

ALOE VERA
Studies have shown this to be effective in the prevention and treatment of radiation burns. The fresh leaf can be cut and the thick juice squeezed onto the affected area. Cold-pressed juice may also be purchased to use as a lotion.

BUCKWHEAT
The leaves of Buckwheat (Fagopyrum esculentum) are an important source of bioflavonoids, especially rutin, and are renowned in the treatment of radiation damage. Take as an infusion. Buckwheat is more commonly known for its grain (the Japanese make Soba noodles from it) and the grain does also contain some bioflavonoids.

KELP
Kelp (Fucus vesiculosis) and other types of brown seaweed are a natural source of iodine (see above). It is also possible that the lignin fibres in kelp and other seaweeds help to remove heavy metals and radiation from the body. Certainly supplements of sodium alginate, extracted from kelp, have been shown to remove radioactive strontium from the bones of laboratory rats. Because kelp is a natural food source, there is no safety limit, and it may be incorporated into the diet or taken as tablets or capsules. It is important to ensure that the kelp you take is sourced away from radiation contaminated areas.

MARIGOLD
Marigold (Calendula officinalis) is a healing and regenerative herb that is useful in the treatment of radiation damage. Internally the infusion is a lymphatic cleanser. Externally the herb is helpful in the treatment of radiation burns. See the entry in the Herbal Remedies section for further information.

MISO
Miso is a traditional Japanese food prepared from soya beans, cereals and sea salt. It is used as a base for soups and sauces, and contains many nutrients. Dr Akizuki based at a hospital in Nagasaki at the time of the bomb believes that the intake of Miso daily as part of a traditional Japanese diet was very helpful in recovery. Although not a cure, Miso certainly does provide a wide range of nutrients in a form very readily assimilated by the body. This and

the fact that it has been renowned in traditional Chinese medicine as 'strengthening to the blood', may indicate why it is so helpful.

SIBERIAN GINSENG (ELEUTHEROCOCCUS SENTICOSUS):
This herb is used in traditional Chinese medicine to increase immune function, and to encourage resistance to free radical toxins and viruses. Studies in China have shown it to be effective in assisting recovery from radiation injury and to enable patients to tolerate higher doses of radiation therapy.
Dosage: 1/4 teaspoon powdered root in boiling water once a day, or 150mg capsule three times daily.

Homœopathic Remedies
Dr Grimmer, writing at the height of the cold war recommended carrying Arnica 30 and Phosphorus 30. He suggested they would be helpful to any survivor not too close to the centre of an atomic explosion. Arnica should be taken for the immediate effects such as shock and bruising. This should be followed after half an hour by Phosphorus which he states, "meets the destructive effects produced on the capillary circulation and later on the blood elements as well. Phosphorus is a remedy for deep burns as well as for ulcerations of a serious nature." (Reported on the website of the National Centre for Homeopathy, USA. www.homeopathic.org)
This is still good advice for immediate action, then follow up with a more specific protocol as outlined below.
The approach for treating the after effects of radiation is similar to that already described in the section Finding the Right Homœopathic Remedy on page 34. If there is an obvious constitutional remedy based on psychological and physical symptoms then prescribe it. The constitutional remedy may be prescribed alongside the more specific recommendations following.

FOR RADIATION SICKNESS
The most commonly prescribed remedies for the nausea associated with radiation sickness are:

Arsenicum: Nausea, retching and vomiting after eating and drinking. Utter prostration. Extremely anxious and fearful. Restless.

Nux vomica: Most common remedy. Violent vomiting. Intense nausea slightly relieved after vomiting.

Phosphorus: Empty feeling in stomach. Nausea. Craves cold drinks which are vomited in a little while. Anxious and melancholic.

FOR EFFECTS OF RADIATION FALL-OUT

The type of radiation caused by different scenarios does vary, and the best results will be obtained by taking the remedy specific to the cause. For example, those exposed to depleted uranium from US missiles should take Depleted Uranium in potency.

Many types of radiation fallout contain a cocktail of radioactive components. Practitioners visiting Russia following the Chernobyl nuclear power station disaster were prescribed Strontium / Caesium/ Radium bromide 30 to take once a week.

The fallout from a nuclear attack is likely to contain plutonium, so Plutonium in potency would be appropriate following exposure to fallout from a nuclear bomb.

As soon as you know what the cocktail of radiation particles you are dealing with contains, then it is advisable to get that made up into a combination remedy by your homœopathic pharmacy. If the exact components are not known, or for immediate use, the following combination remedy has been found to be useful by homœopaths for both effects on the organism and helping to prevent ongoing genetic effects Cobalt / Radium bromide / X-Ray. This should be taken in the 30C potency once a week for several weeks.

PART II

HOW TO MAKE AND USE NATURAL REMEDIES

HERBAL
REMEDIES

Herbs are one of our most ancient forms of medicine. Before drugs, before hospitals, before doctors, before chemist shops, people had worked out which herbs could be used to treat which illnesses. In many parts of the world, herbs are still the most commonly used type of medicine.

Every society has its herbal tradition. In the developed world we nearly lost that knowledge, but a few enlightened and dedicated individuals kept it alive, until its worth was again recognised more widely. If hospitals were not functional, doctors incapacitated and pharmacies closed, there would still be herbs growing.

The herbs referred to in this book have been chosen because they are the most useful for first-aid situations. You can save lives by using herbs for their antimicrobial and anti-inflammatory properties. This fact was utilised during the war in former Yugoslavia in the 1990s, where certain British soldiers were trained to recognise and use specific herbs for emergency situations.

Many of the most versatile medicinal herbs grow just about everywhere in Europe and North America, including inner cities, and have a long growing season. Loose herbs, tinctures and herbal creams can also be readily purchased in health food shops and pharmacies. In other parts of the world, local knowledge should be accessed to find out about the most effective native herbal medicines; although certain, particularly useful herbal medicines such as Echinacea, Marigold and Tea Tree Oil could also be imported.

Those of us lucky enough to have a garden, can easily grow sufficient for a family's use of herbs such as Comfrey, Lemon Balm, Marigold, St John's Wort and Thyme. Ideally, grow the herbs organically, without adding chemical fertilisers, pesticides, etc. Most herbs grow readily on relatively infertile soil and do not need much feeding anyway. By growing on a small scale, you should be able to hand weed the area until the plant is established. It is in the nature of most herbs to be fairly pest resistant, so pesticides should not be necessary.

Once you have a successful crop you can save the seeds for future years, thus reducing dependence on commercial growers. With most herbs, Marigold is a good example, you simply wait for the flowers to develop and die off, and then on a dry day collect a few seed heads in a brown paper bag. Store them somewhere dry over the winter and then sow in seed trays in the spring. Many of the Labiatae family, eg. Sage, Thyme, and other herbs, can also be reproduced by planting cuttings.

If you do not have a garden, a useful supply of a few herbs could be grown in tubs on a patio, balcony or even in a window box. Herbs can also be grown indoors in pots, either in a sunny room, or by using 'daylight' simulating light bulbs to provide sufficient light.

A number of herbs are known as 'pioneer plants', that is they grow readily on waste ground, or in 'wild zones' that can be found in most large parks and nature reserves these days. Whilst herbs are obviously best cultivated in commercial quantities in the countryside; there is an argument that plants tough enough to survive city conditions may actually be more beneficial for people that live in the city. Next time you are out walking in your local area, see how many different herbs you can spot, and note the type of conditions where they are growing.

Obviously plants growing along a main road, whether in the countryside or the city, are best avoided because of the high amounts of lead and other pollutants they may contain. Although even in this case, if you gather the young shoots in the spring, and avoid the mature plant and roots, you can minimise the amount of undesired pollutants. Similarly, avoid plants growing at the base of trees in urban areas if they are evidently favoured spots for dogs to urinate and defecate. Also check that there are no signs of recent spraying with weed killer.

It is important with wasteland to check that the area has not been used as a dump for toxic waste; ask locally if there is any doubt. Plants can be used to decontaminate land; sunflowers for example are being used to decontaminate radioactive soil. However, the initial plants will need to be regularly harvested and incinerated, and a system of measurement set up to determine how successful the process is.

If you do wild-craft herbs, then there are a few simple guidelines to follow:
* Check your source for obvious pollutants (see above).
* Gather only enough for your immediate use.
* Never deplete the whole stock; you or somebody else may need more later.

- Do not dig up the roots, this will mean that the plant will not be available for others or future use. It is also illegal to dig up any wild plants in the UK due to conservation issues.
- Be certain that you are collecting the right species. Some plants that look similar to useful herbs may be poisonous, this is especially true of plants from the Umbelliferae family. Use a field guide and if you are not absolutely certain don't risk it. "The Medicinal Flora", by Julian Barker, is recommended (see Further Reading).

Useful First-Aid Medicinal Herbs That Can Be Wild-Crafted or Cultivated in a Small Garden or Allotment
(For usage see the Herbal Remedy/Materia Medica section)
Arnica, Chamomile, Comfrey, Echinacea, Garlic, Lemon Balm, Mallow, Marigold (Calendula), Marshmallow, Plantain, St Johns Wort, Thyme, Yarrow

USING HERBAL REMEDIES

INFUSIONS

An infusion is another word for a tea. Infusions can be taken internally either hot or cold. Hot infusions are the more usual way to take herbs and will encourage sweating, so use for treating flu, fevers, etc. Cold infusions tend to be more diuretic.

Make an infusion as you would a tea: pour boiling water on to the herb and leave it to draw for a few minutes, and then strain and drink. Always cover the pot or cup whilst it is infusing to keep in the volatile oils. You may add honey or lemon to improve the flavour, although part of the action of bitter herbs is in their taste in the mouth, so don't overdo the sweetness.

A standard dosage for fresh herbs is to use two heaped teaspoons of the cut herb per cupful of boiling water. Allow it to stand for 7-10 minutes and then strain and drink. If using dried herbs, use one heaped teaspoon of herb per cupful of water. For most complaints, infusions are taken three times a day.

For children 7-12 years halve the adult dosage. For children 2-6 years use a quarter. Only very mild herbs, eg. Marshmallow and Chamomile should be used for infants under 2 years, and then use only 1-2 teaspoonfuls of infusion as a dose.

Infusions can also be used externally as a simple lotion. Follow the same directions above, and when cool apply with cotton wool or a clean cloth. Marigold for example can be used in this way as an effective antiseptic and healing wash for wounds.

DECOCTIONS

When using the woody or fibrous parts of a plant, such as barks, roots and berries, it will be necessary to simmer the herb to extract the active constituents. Place the herb or mixture of herbs in a saucepan (not aluminium or chipped enamel), add water, cover and simmer for 10 minutes. Then strain and drink.

Use a heaped tablespoonful of dried herb to 500ml (1 pint) of water, or a heaped teaspoon of herb to a cupful of water, as a standard dose. The water may need to be topped up if much steam escapes.

The decoction can be kept cool for a day or two and taken a glass at a time. For most complaints, decoctions are usually taken three times a day. For childrens' dosage see Infusions above.

CAPSULES

Capsules may be preferable for some herbs with an unpleasant taste, and are convenient to carry around. The herb material will need to be finely ground to a powder if you are going to fill your own capsules. Pour the powdered herb into a small dish, separate the 2 halves of the capsule case and slide them together through the powder, scooping it into the capsule. Then fit together the 2 halves of the capsule. Capsules are available that are made from animal gelatin or vegetable starch.

TINCTURES

A tincture is an extraction of a herb using (usually) alcohol and water. The alcohol acts as a preservative, and so it means that the tincture will stay fresh for several months. It is also a very convenient way to take herbs, as you simply take a few drops in water, and do not need to make an infusion every time. Tinctures may also be used externally, eg. diluted Marigold tincture is an excellent lotion for healing cuts and wounds.

Different countries have different pharmacopoeias, which may recommend varying quantities of alcohol to use and varying ratios of herb to liquid, but the following directions will show you how to make a tincture in your home, that will be effective at the standard dosages given.

EQUIPMENT:
Sealable jars (eg. jam jars), measuring jug, fine mesh cloth (muslin, old tights), unbleached coffee filter, dark glass bottles and lids, labels.

INGREDIENTS:
Fresh herb material. Use a third the quantity of dried herb if
        fresh is unavailable.
Water. Use bottled spring, distilled or filtered and boiled water.
Alcohol. 100% proof ethanol is used commercially, but high
        proof vodka is an acceptable and more readily available
        alternative.

METHOD:
1. Tightly pack a sealable jar, with finely chopped fresh herb.
2. Combine one third alcohol and two thirds water, sufficient to fill the jar (remember the herb will take up more than half the volume of the jar).
3. Pour the liquid into the jar, taking care to completely immerse the herb.

4. Seal the jar and store for 2 weeks out of direct sunlight. Shake the jar every day or two.
5. Strain the mixture through a fine cloth and then filter through an unbleached coffee filter.
6. Pour into a dark glass bottle. Label clearly with the name of the herb and date, and store in a cool place out of direct sunlight.

DOSAGE:
The standard dosage for a tincture when treating chonic disease is between 2ml and 4ml taken in a wine glass of water 3 times a day. 1ml is approx 25 drops. A standard teaspoon is 4ml. For children 2-12 do not use more than 1ml. For infants under 2 years use 5 drops and use only the mild herbs.

When treating first-aid situations and serious acutes, then both the dosage and frequency of giving may be much higher. 15ml every 30 minutes to 2 hours may be required. Again, for children 2-12 give a quarter or less of the dose, and for infants under 2 years do not give more than 0.5ml (approx 10 drops) and only use mild herbs. Always bear in mind that tinctures contain alcohol, and be aware of the quantity taken.

If you add the tincture to hot water, some of the alcohol will evaporate off, which you may find preferable.

COMPRESSES

A compress is an external application that is excellent for soothing inflammation and relieving pain. A compress uses an infusion or decoction of herbs, or essential oils diluted in water. Compresses are usually most effective when using hot water, but if the affected part already feels too hot, a cold compress may be preferable, made by cooling and adding ice to the infusion.

COMPRESS EQUIPMENT:
Basin, towel, hot water, piece of cotton cloth, eg. lint or clean flannel.

COMPRESS METHOD:
Pour infusion into basin, ensuring it is still warm but not too hot so as to scald the skin. Soak cloth in infusion, squeeze out excess fluid and then place directly over area to treat. Wrap a towel around the area and keep it warm. A sheet of cling film (plastic wrap) may be wrapped around the towel, and a hot water bottle may be used to keep the part warm. When the compress cools down the process may be repeated.

This method is an ideal way to use essential oils. Simply add 4-5 drops of essential oil to the hot water and then proceed as for an infusion. Do not let cling film come into contact with essential oils.

HERBS COMMONLY USED FOR COMPRESSES:
Chamomile, Comfrey, Marigold, Marshmallow, Plantain, Slippery Elm,

POULTICES

The action of a poultice is similar to that of a compress, but instead of using a liquid extract, the actual plant material is used. Poultices are an excellent way of treating injuries, eg. sprains, bruising, fractures and for drawing pus out of the skin.

POULTICE EQUIPMENT:
Muslin bag or piece of clean cloth (men's handkerchief), rolling pin, a little vegetable oil, clingfilm (plastic wrap).

POULTICE METHOD:
Place fresh herb in a muslin bag or fold into a cotton cloth. Break herb down to release the juices using a rolling pin. If using dried herb, you will need to mash thoroughly with a little honey or vegetable oil to make a paste. Apply a little vaseline or vegetable oil to the skin to make the poultice easier to remove, and then place/spread the herb over the area. If the skin is broken use a layer of sterile lint between the herb and the skin. Immediately cover the area with clingfilm or a clean cloth and a bandage, and keep warm. Leave on for 3-4 hours.

HERBS COMMONLY USED FOR POULTICES:
Cabbage, raw (to draw pus, inflammation); Comfrey (fractures, strains, ulcers); Marigold (inflammation, skin infections); Marshmallow (to draw pus), Potato, grated raw (bruises), Slippery Elm (to draw pus, boils, abscesses).

MACERATED OILS

Infused, or macerated oils contain the active components of a herb in a vegetable oil base. They are made by saturating the herb with oil and then allowing the properties of the herb to infuse into the oil. The oil can then be used as a massage oil, rub, bath oil, or used as a base for an ointment or cream.

Suitable base oils include Almond, Sunflower and Olive. Traditionally clarified butter or animal fat was used. Once made, a macerated oil should keep for up to a year.

Sun Method of Making a Macerated Oil
This is a relatively slow method of making a macerated oil but the end result is of excellent quality. It is best to use fresh herbs for this method.

This method may also be used for making a herb vinegar, simply replace the oil with cider or white wine vinegar.

EQUIPMENT:
Measuring jug, sealable jar, mesh strainer, bottle.

DIRECTIONS:
1. Pack a sealable jar with finely chopped fresh herb.
2. Cover the herb with the oil. It is important to completely cover the herb with oil to exclude contamination.
3. Seal the jar and leave in direct sunlight for 2 weeks. Shake daily.
4. Strain and repeat with fresh plant material. Leave for another 2 weeks, shaking daily.
5. Strain and pour into bottle. Label with name and date.

Quick Kitchen Method of Making a Macerated Oil
This is a faster method, and is suitable for fresh or dried herbs.

EQUIPMENT:
Measuring jug, heatproof container/bowl, saucepan, mesh strainer, bottle.

INGREDIENTS:
50-75g (2-3oz) dried herb
or 75-100g (3-4oz) fresh herb
300ml (1/2 pint) vegetable oil

DIRECTIONS:
1. Place half the quantity of herb in a bowl and pour on the oil.
2. Cover the bowl if possible and place over a pan of boiling water. Simmer for 2 hours.
3. Strain the herb off and repeat the process using the second amount of plant material.
4. When cooled slightly, strain and pour into a bottle. If using fresh herb, a watery green liquid may appear at the bottom of the oil when it settles. This liquid needs to be separated off and discarded as it may deteriorate and contaminate the oil. Label bottle with name and date.

HERBS SUITABLE FOR MAKING MACERATED OIL:
Calendula, Comfrey, Garlic, St. John's Wort, Thyme

OINTMENTS

Salves and ointments are easy to make and an excellent way of using herbs on the skin. They are oily in nature and will form a soothing, protective layer on the skin. They are ideal for treating infants, elderly people, bruises and sprains, and areas of delicate skin, eg. lips. They may also be used for treating cuts, sores and minor burns. Because they encourage the skin to retain heat and moisture, ointments should not be used in hot, inflamed or weepy skin conditions.

Some herbs may work best in combination, eg. Marigold and St John's Wort (known as Hypericum and Calendula or Hypercal) ointment is an excellent antiseptic for cuts, abrasions and sores. Simply combine the herbs to make up the total quantity required.

Vaseline Based Ointment

The simplest way of making an ointment is by using Vaseline (petroleum jelly) as a base. Although this has the disadvantage of being inorganic, it has the advantages of being easy to use and staying a long time on the skin.

EQUIPMENT FOR VASELINE BASED OINTMENT:
Small saucepan, wire-mesh strainer or fine mesh cloth (muslin, clean old tights, etc.), jar with lid.

INGREDIENTS:

200g Vaseline

50g fresh herb, eg. Comfrey, Marigold

or 25g dried herb

METHOD FOR VASELINE BASED OINTMENT:

1. Melt Vaseline in small saucepan.
2. Add herb, bring to boil, and simmer very gently for 15 minutes stirring constantly.
3. Strain, carefully squeezing out all the liquid.
4. Pour liquid into jar and label with name and date.

Oil and Wax Based Ointment

Various vegetable oils, eg. almond, olive, sunflower and wheatgerm, can be used to make an ointment, which will be thickened with wax. Any wax can be used, eg. candle wax, paraffin wax, but beeswax is ideal as it brings its own healing properties. The herb content can be provided by either adding tinctures to the ointment base, or by using a macerated oil as the vegetable oil. Essential oils may also be added to the base.

EQUIPMENT FOR OIL AND WAX OINTMENT:
Heatproof bowl, saucepan of boiling water, jar with lid.

INGREDIENTS FOR APPROX 100G OINTMENT:

60ml (4 tablespoons) vegetable or macerated oil

8g (2 teaspoons) wax, beeswax if possible (granules or grated)

10ml (2 1/2 teaspoons) required tincture (may not be necessary if using macerated oil)

METHOD FOR OIL AND WAX OINTMENT:

1. Heat the wax and oil in a bowl over a saucepan of boiling water until the wax has melted.
2. Remove from the heat and add the tincture. Stir gently.
3. Allow to cool slightly before pouring into jar. Label with name and date.

HERBS SUITABLE FOR MAKING OINTMENTS:

For Healing the Skin, Wounds and Preventing and Treating Infection: Echinacea, Lavender Oil, Marigold, Plantain, St John's Wort, Tea Tree Oil

For Muscles, Joints, Broken Bones and Bruising: Arnica, Comfrey, Lavender Oil, Marigold

For Chest Rubs/Inhalations: Tea Tree Oil, Thyme

HOMŒOPATHIC REMEDIES

Homœopathic remedies can transform your health in the most remarkable way. They also have an exceptional record in the treatment of serious acute and epidemic diseases, eg. smallpox, typhoid, cholera. Because they act on your vital or energetic body, and not directly on your physical or bio-chemical body, they can work incredibly quickly and effectively. However, the disadvantage can be that although in some situations self treatment is straightforward, in others, skill and accuracy is needed to determine which is the correct remedy and the best potency.

Precision is also needed in the making of homœopathic remedies, and whilst it is possible to make some of your own remedies (see below), needing to use homœopathic pharmacies, at least for the source material of the more exotic remedies, is likely. However, once you have the remedy in base (mother) tincture form you can reproduce the remedy for just about forever, which also illustrates how environmentally sustainable homœopathy is.

HOW TO MAKE HOMŒOPATHIC REMEDIES

Homœopathic remedies can be made from almost anything, including: minerals, plants, animal substances, eg. bee venom, and also non-material 'radiations', eg. sunlight. The source material of some commonly used remedies is given in the Remedy section of this book.

The first step in making most homœopathic remedies is to produce a base tincture, known as a 'mother tincture' (follow the directions in the Herbal section to make a tincture). Some plants, eg. resins, as well as most minerals are not readily soluble in alcohol and have to be prepared first by grinding (triturating) with an inert powder (traditionally lactose, or milk sugar, but you could use sucrose, or cane sugar, if that's all that was available). After this they become soluble and a tincture can be prepared in the same way as for alcohol-soluble plants.

A homœopathic pharmacopoeia will give varying precise directions for each remedy and each potency, but the following directions will produce a dynamic and effective remedy that you can make and use in your own home or clinic. The method described is known as the Korsakov method and has been used by homœopathic pharmacies in France and Belgium for many years.

Making a 6C Potency

EQUIPMENT:
One small (20ml would be ideal) sterile glass vial or bottle with stopper/lid, mother tincture, alcohol (pure 'medical' alcohol or vodka).

METHOD:
1. To make a 1C potency add 2 drops of mother tincture to the small glass bottle. Carefully add 10ml of alcohol. Secure the lid.
2. Hold the bottle firmly in one hand and bang it repeatedly (succussion) against the palm of the other hand (or on a desk or book) for 100 bangs (about one minute).
3. Pour out the contents of the bottle, leaving droplets on the inside of the glass. The droplets are sufficient to medicate the next potency. Add another 10ml of alcohol to the bottle. Repeat the succussion process for a further 100 bangs.
4. Repeat the process of dilution and succussion another 4 times (6 in total) and the resulting potency is known as a 6C.

Higher Potencies

If the process is repeated 30 times, the remedy would be referred to as a 30C potency: this is a potency frequently used in treating acute situations. It is also possible to make 200C remedies using this method or even 1000C (1M).

Medicating Pills

The liquid potencies can be taken by adding one drop to a small amount of water and drinking. Or add 3-4 drops of the liquid potency to a small bottle of lactose carrier pills, replace the lid, and turn the bottle upside down for a few seconds. The pills are then ready to use.

To make larger quantities of remedies you can simply scale up the process; the directions given are sufficient for about 50 bottles of pills.

FINDING THE RIGHT HOMŒOPATHIC REMEDY

A homœopathic remedy is usually chosen by matching the most appropriate remedy 'picture' to that of the sufferer. Observe and note as many physical and emotional symptoms of the sufferer as you can, and then use these as clues to find the right remedy (the 'similimum').

In first-aid situations, a match between the physical symptoms of the patient, and the physical indications for the remedy will usually suffice. For example, after a physical injury nearly everyone will benefit from a dose of the main first-aid remedy Arnica.

In other situations, if the remedy itself has a strong emotional or 'personality' picture, this should be the guiding factor and not necessarily the physical indications. For example, if a child with diarrhoea becomes unusually weepy and clingy give him the remedy Pulsatilla whatever the physical type of diarrhoea he has. (Pulsatilla is a remedy for people who become weepy, clingy and demanding when unwell).

So, ask the sufferer as many questions as you can think of directly relevant to their ailment, then note how the patient is behaving, and then check those against the indications in the Remedy section of this book.

The scope of this book is to cover emergencies and thus the focus is on those remedies that cover first-aid, acute and epidemic situations. For this reason many of the remedies suggested are recommended as a protocol, ie. in a given situation try this remedy or this series of remedies.

Using a protocol is particularly appropriate where the remedies known as nosodes are recommended or when treating things such as radiation exposure. This is because during an epidemic of a contagious disease, or following exposure to chemical or radiation attack, most people affected will display a similar set of symptoms; the protocol remedy is the similimum for the exposure, not necessarily the individual. The most specific remedy indicated for a particular epidemic is known in homœopathy as the genus epidemicus. An American organisation, the National Centre for Homeopathy, has added a place to its website with the intention of posting the genus epidemicus for public access when required. See www.homeopathic.org

Experienced homœopaths may use the protocol advised here and also, if there is a clear constitutional picture for an individual, prescribe the constitutional remedy as well. Indeed, the best results may well come from giving an individual the relevant protocol and also their constitutional remedy to take. For example, if a woman displaying clear Sepia symptoms has reason to believe she may have been subjected to anthrax spores then give her Anthracinum 30 once a week and also a dose of Sepia in an appropriate potency as a constitutional remedy.

DOSAGE

The most common potency used for treating acute and first-aid situations is the 30th potency (30C or 30 centesimal). Other potencies that you find readily available, or can make, are 6C and 200C. Generally speaking, the more severe the symptoms then the higher the potency that you take; and the higher the potency then the less frequently you take the remedy.

It can seem bizarre at first, to those new to energetic medicine, that the more dilute the substance is, the higher and more dynamic the potency is. If this is an issue then it is important to appreciate that as well as dilution, the succussion process is integral to making a homœopathic remedy, and so a higher potency is both more refined and has had more energy input than a lower potency.

When the symptoms are very acute, a 6C potency can be given every one or two hours until things improve. A 30 potency can be given three or four times a day or, if the symptoms are quite extreme, one or two doses only of a 200 potency may be given. For example, Arnica 6 can be given repeatedly over several days for bruising, aches and pains. When the injury involves some shock to the body use a few doses of Arnica 30 over three or four days. Arnica 200 would be much more effective if the person is in a severe state of shock after an accident, or following the profound physical experience of childbirth. One or two doses should be sufficient. The following chart may help to make things clearer, although it is only a guideline.

	MINOR AILMENTS Eg. sprains & strains, colds	ACUTE Eg. flu, fevers, following accidents and injuries	VERY SERIOUS Eg. head injury, more serious accidents, burns, haemorrhage	PREVENTION
6 or 6x	One three times a day for up to 10 days.	One every 2 to 4 hours. Reduce frequency as symptoms improve.		
30	One morning and night for up to 5 days.	One every 4 hours for one day only. Then 1 or 2 a day for 3 to 5 days, stop if symptoms improve.	One every 2-4 hours for 3 or 4 days. Then 2 a day until symptoms improve.	One dose once or twice a week.
200			One dose only. Repeat only if symptoms are clearly indicated. No more than 3 doses in total.	

HOW TO TAKE HOMŒOPATHIC REMEDIES

Homœopathic remedies are manufactured as tablets, granules, powders or liquids. Tablets are the most easily managed and the most usual form. One tablet constitutes one dose. This is more than adequate to initiate a healing response, and you will not get a stronger effect by taking a larger number of tablets.

Unlike herbs, ideally it is best not to combine homœopathic remedies at any one time. It is preferable to find the one remedy that fits the symptoms best and take that, then if the symptoms change try a different remedy. On those occasions when you may need to take more than one remedy, take them at different times of the day or if possible on different days of the week. For example if you are taking treatment for a back injury and you also need to take a preventative remedy during an outbreak of smallpox, then take one for the back problem in the morning and the preventative one (eg. Variolinum) in the evening.

Homœopathic tablets (or as liquid) are taken by placing one under the tongue and allowing it to dissolve. The mouth needs to be clean of any other substances, so do not eat, drink, smoke or brush your teeth for 15 minutes or so before and after taking a remedy.

For infants a tablet may be crushed between two clean teaspoons and then tipped into the mouth, or give a liquid dose. This method may also be used if treating someone who is unconscious.

Try not to handle the remedies, but shake one dose into the lid of the bottle and then tip it straight into your mouth.

It is advisable to avoid taking coffee and strong smelling substances such as camphor and eucalyptus whilst using a homœopathic treatment, as they may antidote it. No harm will be produced by combining homœopathic with orthodox drugs, although it may mean that the homœopathic remedy does not work so effectively.

Homœopathic remedies should be stored in their original container, away from strong smells and out of the light. Do not expose homœopathic remedies to X-Rays, as this may reduce their effectiveness; if necessary ask airport officials to look at them rather than having them X-Rayed with your luggage.

Speed of Remedy Action

In a very acute or first-aid situation the right homœopathic remedy should work very quickly, with the patient experiencing relief from the most urgent and painful symptoms within minutes of taking the remedy. Good examples of this that spring to mind are the relief from pain experienced within a couple of minutes of taking Hypericum after someone slamming a car door on their finger; and an infant's very high temperature dropping to less dangerous levels minutes after administering Belladonna.

These are dramatic situations where it is very clear that the correct remedy was given. In less acute situations the remedy may take longer to achieve noticeable results, although generally speaking in any non-chronic illness some improvement should be felt within a few hours of taking a remedy. There may be an obvious relief of symptoms, or the patient feels 'better in themselves', or they have a deep and refreshing sleep soon after taking the remedy. Chronic conditions, ie. those that the patient has had for months or even years, will usually take longer to cure, and here you need to be guided by an experienced practitioner.

Many illnesses have clear symptoms and respond quickly to the best indicated remedy. If the remedy you first try doesn't work, then check the symptoms against the remedies again, and try a different remedy. Of course some illnesses are complicated and hard to treat, and if at all possible it may be best to seek advice from someone with more experience. However, it is worth bearing in mind that no harm can come from trying a homœopathic remedy - if it is the wrong remedy it simply will not work.

How Long to Take the Remedy?
Once the remedy has showed signs of working, and the symptoms improve, then STOP taking the remedy. If the symptoms return some time after stopping taking the remedy, then repeat the remedy. Some illnesses may require more than one remedy to bring about a cure, the guideline is that if the symptoms change, then select a different remedy that covers the new picture.

PREVENTION
The method of taking a homœopathic remedy to prevent a disease is called homœopathic prophylaxis. There are a number of examples of the efficacy of using homœopathic prophylaxis to prevent contagious diseases in the homœopathic literature. The eminent homœopath Leslie Speight writes of a physician who gave Lathyrus sativa to 82 people who were in close proximity to a polio outbreak, with 12 people being direct contacts, and not one developed the disease. There are also many accounts in current farming journals of homœopathic vets getting excellent results by giving farm animals homœopathic nosodes to prevent common farm diseases.

The method is to choose the remedy, and take a dose just before or following any known contact with a disease.

Sometimes a special type of homœopathic remedy, called a nosode, is used for prophylaxis. Nosodes are actually made from diseased body tissue or discharges such as sputum. Nosodes may be purchased from homœopathic pharmacies, or if that is not a possibility, you could make a nosode following the directions for making homœopathic remedies given above. This could be very useful in a 'state of emergency' situation.

The standard dosage for homœopatic prevention is to give one dose of the 30C potency a week for as long as exposure to the disease continues, ie. for the duration of an outbreak. If the exposure to the disease was a one-off, eg. when giving Ledum to prevent tetanus following a punctured wound, then give one dose of the 30C potency twice a week for three weeks.

Whilst homœopathic prevention can be very effective, there is never any absolute guarantee that you will not get a disease whatever measures you take, because there is always a possibility that you are exceptionally susceptible to a particular disease. Also if your immune system is already compromised then you will be more susceptible to any disease. However, the appropriate remedy given as prophylaxis should mean that you get a milder form of the disease than you would had you not taken it. It should also be noted that conventional immunisation has significant failure rates for certain diseases, eg. polio, cholera.

PART III

THE REMEDIES/ MATERIA MEDICA

HERBAL
REMEDIES

ARNICA

Arnica montana   Family: Compositae
Habitat: Native to Denmark, Southern Scandinavia,
               Germany and East France. Cultivated elsewhere.
Parts Used: Flowers
Collection: When the flowers are fully open in summer.
Actions: Anti-inflammatory

Uses

An exceptionally effective remedy to promote healing of bruises, injuries, contusions, sprains and strains. Apply as a cream or lotion where the skin is not broken. Also useful for rheumatism and neuralgia, especially if following an injury.

As a plant medicine Arnica is only used externally because it is toxic internally; it is also used widely as a homœopathic remedy.

Preparations

Compress
Tincture as lotion or compress
Cream or ointment
Macerated oil
Homœopathic remedy

Safety

External use only. Not to be used on broken skin because it is toxic internally and may be absorbed into the blood stream through broken skin.

BALM, LEMON BALM

Melissa officinalis   Family: Labiatae

Habitat:	Native of Southern Europe but naturalized to Britain, and grows readily.
Parts Used:	Aerial parts
Collection:	Fresh leaves may be picked in early summer. Dried for use throughout the year.
Actions:	Anti-depressive, anti-flatulence, anti-spasmodic, anti-histamine, anti-stress, anti-viral, mild tranquilliser, hypotensive.

Uses

INTERNAL:

A pleasant tasting herbal tea that is an excellent nerve tonic. Used to treat nervousness, insomnia, stress, depression. Useful for post-traumatic stress. Generally lifts the spirits. Headaches, especially tension headaches. Cramping pains and gas in the gut. Indigestion. Tonic to heart and circulatory system, lowers blood pressure. Fevers, especially in children, childhood illnesses. May be safely given to children to help with sleep problems, colic and other digestive problems.

Preparations

Infusion:	Standard infusion.
Tincture:	2-5ml three times a day.

Useful Combinations

For digestive, sleep problems and stress: Chamomile

Safety

Well tolerated and especially suitable for children. Safe to take during pregnancy.

CHAMOMILE, ROMAN & GERMAN

Anthemis nobilis, Chamaemelum nobile (Roman)   Family: Compositae
Matricaria chamomilla, M. recutita (German)   Family: Compositae

Habitat: There are a large number of different types of
              Chamomile, some are different races, others are the
              results of different environments. The two most com-
              monly used medicinally are listed above. Anthemis
              nobilis and Chamomilla recutita can be found through-
              out Europe on wasteland, verges and fallow soil.
Parts Used: Flowers
Collection: Gather flowers between May and August.
Actions: Antispasmodic, analgesic, anti-inflammatory,
              antiseptic, carminative, de-sensitiser, mild seda-
              tive, digestive tonic

Uses

A great calming and anti-inflammatory herb. Both types of
Chamomile share similar therapeutic properties. German Chamomile
is slightly more anti-inflammatory than Roman Chamomile.

INTERNAL:
An immensely versatile and useful herb for both adults and children. Calming and relaxing for anxiety and insomnia. Helps to
reduce fever in childhood illnesses. Promotes white blood cell production so may be taken as a tonic for any inflammatory or infectious condition, eg. flu, earache, etc. Relieves many kinds of painful
digestive complaints including indigestion, gastritis, diarrhoea, gas,
colic, nausea. Period pains. Palpitations. Radiation sickness.

EXTERNAL:
Soothes all manner of inflammations, allergic reactions. Inflamed
eyes. Nappy rash.

Preparations

Infusion: Standard infusion internally or as lotion.
Tincture: 3-5ml three times daily or more frequently in
              extreme situations internally. Externally as lotion or
              compress.
Compress: Strong infusion used hot.
Essential oil
Ointments and creams

Useful combinations

For children: Balm.

Safety

Extremely safe to use for all, including infants.

COMFREY

Symphytum officinale   Family: Boraginaceae
Habitat: Widespread throughout Northern Europe,
               especially in damp places.
Parts Used: Root and leaf.
Collection: Leaves May to August.
               Roots unearth and divide in autumn.
Actions: Astringent-demulcent, expectorant,
               cell regenerator and restorer, wound healing.

Uses

The leaves to be taken internally, both the leaves and root used externally. Contains allantoin which has powerful healing properties both inside and out. It would be helpful to take after any poisoning that caused irritation to the stomach or lungs.

INTERNAL:

Gut problems including gastric and duodenal ulcers, hiatus hernia, ulcerative colitis. Bleeding from stomach, throat, bowel, bladder and lungs. Irritating coughs, dry lung complaints, eg. pleurisy (increases expectoration). Its country name of knitbone indicates its use for mending broken bones (take internally and use externally).

EXTERNAL:

Heals fractures, sprains, strains, pulled muscles, etc. Bruises, scar tissue. Promotes rapid healing of wounds (use carefully for deep wounds as it can promote scar tissue forming over the wound before it has healed deeper down). Ulcers. Burns including radiation burns. Psoriasis. Rheumatic joints.

Preparations:

Infusion: Standard infusion three times a day.
Tincture: Leaf 2-4ml three times a day internally. Externally
            tincture of leaf and root as lotion or compress.
Compress: Crushed root simmered in water for 10 minutes.
Poultice: Bruise leaf or crush fresh root with rolling pin or
            blend in liquidiser.
Macerated oil, cream or ointment

Safety

The root and to a much lesser extent the leaf contains pyrrolizidine alkaloids which in very large doses can cause liver damage. The root to be used externally only. The herb (leaf) may be taken internally for up to 8 weeks at a time. Externally the herb and root are both non-toxic.

ECHINACEA (CONE FLOWER)

Echinacea angustifolia, E. pallida, E. purpurea Family: Compositae

Habitat: Echinacea is native to the USA and can be cultivated in Europe.

Parts Used: Root, rhizome and whole of the plant.

Collection: Aerial parts may be collected July to September when in flower. The roots should be unearthed and divided in the autumn.

Actions: Antimicrobial, antiseptic, anti-inflammatory, tonic, immune-stimulant, lymphatic.

Uses

Known as nature's great antibiotic.

INTERNAL:

One of the most important herbal remedies in the treatment of any kind of infection. It stimulates the 'killer cell' immune response, ie. it promotes the production of white blood cells. Infections such as boils, abscess, septicaemia. Viral illnesses such as flu. Tonsillitis, laryngitis. Candida. Dysentery. Mouthwash for ulcers, gum infections, etc. Bartram refers to its internal use for the successful treatment of cutaneous anthrax.

EXTERNAL:

Ulcers, boils, septic sores and cuts. Apply locally and use internally for more severe infections.

Preparations

Decoction: Standard decoction

Tincture: 1-4ml three times daily internally. For more extreme situations take every 1-2 hours. Externally as lotion or compress.

Cream or ointment

Useful Combinations

Garlic, Thyme

Safety

Generally well tolerated.

GARLIC AND ONION

Allium sativum and Allium cepa   Family: Liliaceae

Habitat: Cultivated throughout the British Isles. Field Garlic
            (*A. oleraceum*) and Wild Onion (*A. vineale*) are the
            native, wild varieties, which have similar therapeu-
            tic properties to the cultivated types but have
            much smaller bulbs and a less pungent flavour.

Part Used: Bulb

Collection: Unearth bulb when leaves begin to wither in
            autumn.

Actions: Antiseptic, anti-viral, anti-fungal, diaphoretic,
            anti-parasitic, hypotensor, antispasmodic, expecto-
            rant.

Uses

Eating raw garlic will help to prevent any contagious disease; it was
used in previous centuries to help prevent plague. Eat a raw, peeled
clove three times a day before meals.

Garlic is useful for treating intestinal worms and any digestive
infection, eg. food poisoning.

Garlic and onion are both excellent for bronchitis, asthma,
cough, whooping cough, colds and flu. Onion is milder than garlic
and more suitable for children and old people.

EXTERNAL:

Apply the juice to prevent and treat infection in wounds, boils,
styes, etc.

Preparations

Fresh garlic clove: Eaten at mealtimes.

Fresh garlic or onion juice (internal): Half to 1 teaspoon in
            honey or water.

Compress: Mash garlic clove on suitable material.

Poultice: Roast whole onion until soft. Cut in half and
            when cool apply to affected area.

LAVENDER (HERB & OIL)

Lavandula officinalis   Family: Labiatae

Habitat: Native to the Mediterranean region and easily cultivated in Northern Europe.
Parts Used: Flowering tops.
Collection: Gather during the summer when in full flower.
Actions: analgesic, antimicrobial, anti-depressant, anti-inflammatory, insecticide, sedative, vulnerary.

Uses

Herb: The infusion may be taken internally for stress, nervousness, panic and exhaustion. Also for cramping pains and cystitis. Period pains. It can relieve palpitations and high blood pressure. Externally the infusion may be used as a lotion for inflamed skin.

Essential Oil: An incredibly versatile oil used wherever soothing, antiseptic and anti-inflammatory properties are needed. Stress, depression, tension, headaches, insomnia, neuralgia, shock, hysteria. Thrush. First-aid including wounds, burns, insect bites. Radiation burns. Lavender is one of the few essential oils that can be applied neat to the skin to treat infection and inflammation, or use as a compress. Add 5-6 drops to a warm bath or blend 2% in a base oil for a massage oil.

Preparations

Infusion: Standard infusion.
Essential Oil:Steam distilled from the flowering tops. Use for massage, baths, inhalations, compresses, douches, etc.
Combinations: Lavender Oil with Tea Tree Oil for antiseptic and soothing properties.

Safety

Generally a safe and mild herb. The essential oil is extremely safe to use.

LIQUORICE

Glycyrrhiza glabra   Family: Leguminosae

Habitat: Native to Asia and naturalised in France. May be cultivated in Britain.

Parts Used: Dried root.

Collection: Unearth roots in late autumn. Clean and dry.

Actions: adrenal agent, anti-inflammatory, antiviral, demulcent, expectorant, hepato-protective, exhibits anti-tumour activity

Uses

Known as 'the Universal herb' because it can be added to many other herbs to buffer (sweeten and soften) their action. It can be used internally to counter the effects of any kind of poisoning whether inhaled or ingested (chemical poisoning). It supports the liver and reduces irritation. Take for any inflammation of the lungs or stomach. Soothes symptoms of food poisoning.

Preparations

Decoction: Standard decoction.

Infusion: Root may be powdered to make a standard infusion

Capsules: Of powdered root.

Tincture: 2-5ml daily or more frequently for extreme situations.

Safety

Not to be taken by those with high blood pressure or during pregnancy.

MARIGOLD, POT MARIGOLD, CALENDULA

Calendula officinalis   Family: Compositae

Habitat: Native to South Europe but readily cultivated in
              Britain in gardens or pots.
Parts Used: Flowers
Collection: Collect the flower tops between June and
              September. Dry carefully.
Actions: Anti-inflammatory, anti-microbial, astringent,
              anti-fungal, menstrual regulator, anti-cancer,
              healing to tissue, immune stimulant,
              uterine stimulant.

Uses

The greatest healing herb of them all. Promotes healing of all tissue
both internal and skin. Antimicrobial so helps prevent infection.

INTERNAL:

Take following surgical operations to promote internal healing.
Gastric and duodenal ulcer. A blood cleanser so take internally
following any infection, blood poisoning or to cleanse the system
after poisoning.

EXTERNAL:

An excellent herb for local skin problems. Any inflammation of
the skin. Wounds, ulcers, bleeding, bruising, minor burns. Eczema.
Nappy rash. Sore nipples. Thrush. Tooth extractions.

Preparations

Infusion: Standard infusion internally or as lotion externally.
Tincture: 1-3ml internal dose. Externally as lotion or compress.
Poultice: Infuse flowers to soften.
Macerated oil
Ointment or cream

Useful Combinations

Antiseptic lotion: Echinacea, St John's Wort, Witch Hazel.

Safety

Not to be taken internally during pregnancy as it has an emme-
nagogue action (stimulates the periods).

49

MARSHMALLOW AND MALLOW

Althaea officinalis and *Malva sylvestris*   Family: Malvaceae

Habitat: Mallow grows widely on roadsides and waste
              ground all over the British Isles. Marshmallow is
              not so common but can be found as its name
              suggests on damp ground.

Parts Used: Mallow - flowers and leaves. Marshmallow - root
              and leaf.

Collection: Mallow - July to September. Marshmallow - leaves
              in summer after flowering. Root unearthed in late
              autumn.

Actions: Mallow - demulcent, anti-inflammatory, expecto-
              rant, laxative. Marshmallow Leaf - demulcent,
              expectorant, diuretic, emollient. Marshmallow
              Root - demulcent, diuretic, emollient, vulnerary.

Uses

INTERNAL:

Mallow and Marshmallow are soothing, anti-inflammatory and provide a protective coating to irritated tissue. Thus they are useful
to soothe tissue after any kind of irritating poisoning or inflammation.

Mallow -   coughs, bronchial irritation, sore throat, gastritis,
              stomach ulcers.

Marshmallow Leaf - bronchitis, respiratory catarrh, irritating
              coughs, cystitis, urinary gravel, urethritis.

Marshmallow Root - all inflammations of the digestive tract,
              ie. mouth, gastritis, peptic ulcer, colitis, enteritis.

EXTERNAL:

Marshmallow Root - Abscesses, boils, ulcers. Especially for
              'drawing' out pus or foreign bodies.

Preparations

Infusion: Standard infusion.

Tincture: 2-5ml daily or more frequently for extreme situations.

Poultice: Powdered root.

Cream or ointment

Safety

Mild and non toxic. Marshmallow is particularly suitable for children.

50

PLANTAIN

Plantago major   Family: Plantaginaceae
Other Varieties: Ribwort plantain *(P. lanceolata)* and Hoary Plantain
(P. media) also share similar therapeutic properties.

Habitat: Common throughout Europe
              especially in grassy areas.
Parts Used: Leaves.
Collection: Leaves throughout summer.
Actions: Anti-histamine, antimicrobial, anti-haemorrhagic,
              astringent, demulcent, diuretic, expectorant, lym-
              phatic, tonic (blood).

Uses

An incredibly versatile herb with healing properties.

INTERNAL:

Expectorant and soothing for coughs. Astringent for diarrhoea,
gastric ulcers, irritable bowel and cystitis . Cooling tea for fevers,
intermittent fevers. Very soothing and appropriate for allergic
reactions and poisoning where there is irritation.

EXTERNAL:

Use as a cool infusion or dilute the tincture, or use as a compress.
Haemorrhoids, wounds, ulcers. Infected skin conditions, wounds
slow to heal. Scalds and burns. The lotion will soothe painful skin
problems: blisters, chicken pox, shingles, etc. Animal and insect
bites and stings. Douche for vaginal thrush. Mouthwash for
toothache, mouth and gum infections.

Preparations

Infusion: Standard infusion.
Tincture: 1-2ml three times a day.
Compress: Bruised fresh leaves applied to the skin.
Ointment: Use shredded leaves.

Safety

Generally well tolerated.

ST JOHN'S WORT

Hypericum perforatum   Family: Hypericaceae
Habitat: Common on grassland, banks and clearings.
Parts Used: Aerial parts.
Collection: Gather when in flower from June to August.
Actions: Anti-inflammatory, astringent,
              antidepressant, nervine, sedative.

Uses

A healing herb that is anti-depressant when taken internally and an excellent antiseptic when used externally.

INTERNAL:

Well known for the treatment of depression. Infusion used to treat anxiety, nervousness, stress, tension, shock. Nervous exhaustion. Post-traumatic stress. Neuralgia, sciatica, spinal concussion. Cramps. There is some evidence that it is protective against the damaging effects of radiation.

EXTERNAL:

Analgesic (relieves pain) as well as antiseptic. Wounds, bruises, varicose veins, piles, sunburn – make an infusion to use as a lotion or dilute the tincture. Use the diluted tincture for burns. Massage macerated oil in for sciatica, neuralgia, shingles. Macerated oil for radiation burns.

Preparations

Infusion: Standard infusion
Tincture: 2-4ml three times a day.
Macerated Oil: In olive oil base for topical use.
Compress: Infusion for wounds, etc.
Cream or ointment

Useful Combinations

With Marigold for external use as a healing antiseptic in tincture or ointment.

Safety

Not suitable internally for severe depression. Internal use may react with prescribed drugs, so if on medication consult a practitioner before use.

SLIPPERY ELM

Ulmus fulva   Family: Ulmaceae
Habitat: Abundant throughout North America.
Parts Used: The bark is peeled off then dried.
Collection: The bark is stripped off the trunk
              during the spring.
Actions: Emollient, expectorant, demulcent, nutrient.

Uses

A soothing herb that protects mucous membranes by covering them with a coat of mucilage.

INTERNAL:
Remarkable healing properties for any irritation of the digestive tract: gastritis, mucous colitis, enteritis, gastric or duodenal ulcer, dyspepsia, diarrhoea, etc. One of the most useful herbs to treat diarrhoea from food poisoning. Protects gastric mucosa from too much acid. Excellent in debility and convalescence; especially for infants or the elderly. Bronchitis, pleurisy. Would soothe the throat and gut against irritant poisons.

EXTERNAL:
As an anti-inflammatory poultice for wounds, boils, ulcers, burns and any inflammation.

Preparations

Powder: Add half a teaspoon to a cup and mix to a paste
           with a little cold water. Top up with boiling water
           or milk, stirring steadily. Drink before meals for
           acid conditions. Take every 2 hours as a nutritional
           food during convalescence.
Poultice: Mix 1-2 teaspoons of powder to a paste with
           boiling water.

Useful Combinations

With Marshmallow for gastric complaints. With Marshmallow for a 'drawing' poultice (to remove pus or foreign bodies).

Safety

A mild and nutritious herb with no known precautions or contraindications.

TEA TREE OIL

Melaleuca alternifolia   Family: Myrtaceae

Habitat: A tree native to Australia.
Collection: Steam distilled from the leaves
              and twigs of the tree.
Actions: Antiseptic, antibiotic, antifungal, antiviral,
              stimulant, immuno-stimulant, analgesic (mild).

Uses

An extremely effective antimicrobial oil.

Will combat many kinds of bacterial, fungal, or viral infection. It is antiseptic and also stimulates the production of white blood cells and thus the immune response. Colds, coughs and flus (inhalations). Cystitis, genital infections. Athlete's foot, thrush, ringworm. First aid use in boils, wounds, cuts and burns. Insect bites and stings (dab on neat).

Preparations

Use in massage oils, baths, inhalations, compresses, creams, mouthwashes or for small areas dab on neat.

Safety

External use only, toxic internally.

THYME (HERB & OIL)

Thymus vulgaris   Family: Labiatae

Habitat: Garden Thyme (*Thymus vulgaris*) is native to
               Mediterranean Europe and is cultivated
               throughout the world. Wild Thyme (*T. praecox*)
               and Large Leaved Thyme (*T. pulegioides*) are native
               to Britain where they grow on dry grassland.
               All varieties of Thyme share similar therapeutic
               properties although *T. vulgaris* is the most aromatic.

Parts Used: Aerial parts.

Collection: Collect flowering tops and strip leaves off branches
               from June to August.

Actions: Antimicrobial, antioxidant, anti-fungal,
               anti-spasmodic, anti-flatulent, expectorant.

Uses

An effective antimicrobial herb that also stimulates the immune
response.

INTERNAL:

Thyme has a special affinity for the respiratory system and will
relieve many conditions including coughs, bronchitis, whooping
cough, bronchitis, asthma. Colds and flus. Sinusitis. Streptococcal
infections. Sore throat, tonsillitis, laryngitis, gingivitis. Worms.
Digestive tonic; dyspepsia, flatulence. Antimicrobial properties
useful for diarrhoea and dysentery.

EXTERNAL:

Infected wounds, scabies. Fungal infections. Make a strong infusion to use as a simple lotion or use the tincture or essential oil.

Preparations

Infusion: Standard infusion.

Tincture: 2-4ml three times a day.

Compress: Strong infusion for external use,
                also for mouthwash.

Essential Oil: Excellent for external application in a massage
                base or inhalations.

Safety

Avoid internal use in therapeutic doses during pregnancy.

YARROW

Achillea millefolium   Family: Compositae

Habitat: A freely growing wild flower. Likes sun or partial shade. Especially common along roadsides and paths.

Parts Used: Aerial parts.

Collection: Whole of the part above ground when in flower (June-September).

Actions: Antiseptic, astringent, diuretic, hypotensive.

Uses

A useful herb for reducing fevers and stopping haemorrhage.

INTERNAL:

A classic remedy for helping the body to deal with fevers. Colds and flu. Malarial fever. Childhood illnesses, eg. measles, chickenpox. Lowers blood pressure. Digestive tonic. Will relieve diarrhoea and dysentery. Cystitis. Take internally for internal haemorrhage.

EXTERNAL:

Use an infusion to stem blood loss and promote healing of wounds. Nosebleeds.

Preparations:

Infusion: Standard infusion.

Tincture: 2-4ml three times a day.

Poultice: Fresh leaf.

Safety

Excessive doses may cause headaches. Do not use during pregnancy. External use may cause phototoxicity so do not go out into strong sunlight after applying.

HOMŒOPATHIC REMEDIES

ACONITE   ACONITUM NAPELLUS
Common Name: Monkshood
Made From: Potentised fresh plant tincture.

Mental & General
Symptoms come on quickly, violently and intensely. Feeling will
die any minute. Very useful at the beginning of a high fever or
inflammation. Give following any bad fright or shock. In high
potency - any symptom that dates from an intensely frightening
experience, eg. an assault, bombing, car crash, earthquake, etc.
Not usually sustained fear, which is Stramonium. Childhood illnesses. Feeling as if going down with something. The person is
restless, anxious and fearful. Shock. Nightmares. Expects to die
any minute.

Physical
Head:	Heavy and hot. Headache with fever. Feels burst- ing.
Eyes:	Conjunctivitis.
Stomach:	Intense thirst. Violent vomiting.
Abdomen:	Colic. Bloody stools. Dysentery.
Respiratory:	Hoarse, dry, painful cough. Croup. Laryngitis.
Fever:	Chills alternating with heat. High fever. Develops after exposure to a cold wind.
Worse For:	Fright, shock, night, exposure to cold.
Compare:	Belladonna, Opium, Stramonium.

ANT TART ANTIMONIUM TARTARICUM

Common Name: Tartar emetic
Made From: Trituration and solution of tartrate of antimony
and potash.

Mental & General

A remedy for diseases affecting the lungs with a great accumulation of mucus. Breathing becomes difficult and there is rattling in the chest. The heart and circulation become impeded. The patient becomes increasingly weak and drowsy. Delirium. The stomach may also be affected with much nausea and violent vomiting which exhausts the patient. An important remedy for childhood illnesses especially measles. Early stages of smallpox.

Physical

Stomach: Craves acid foods. Nausea comes in waves. Forceful vomiting followed by exhaustion. Violent retching.
Respiratory: Loose, rattling cough. Chest is full of mucus but less and less can be raised. Breathing becomes very difficult. Must sit up to breathe. Cough with vomiting. Bronchitis, pneumonia, whooping cough, asthma. Asphyxia neonatorum.
Fever: Cold clammy sweat.
Worse For: Warmth. Lying down. Sour food. Milk.

APIS APIS MELLIFICA

Common Name: Honey Bee
Made From: Potentised tincture of animal including sting.

Mental & General

Symptoms are very painful and with marked swelling and shiny redness. Pains are sudden and burning, stinging, prickling or like hot needles. Puffy swellings. Water retention. May shriek suddenly with pain. Classic allergic reaction, especially to insect bites and stings. They are very fussy, restless and hard to please. Always busy, just like a bee. Jealous. Awkward - drops things.

Physical

Head: Stabbing pains. Meningitis. Boring of the head backward in pillow, or rolling of head from side to side with brain inflammation.
Eyes: Puffy or red, swollen lids. Hot tears. Conjunctivitis. Styes. Corneal ulcers.
Throat: Throat sore and swollen, swallowing painful. Tonsillitis.

Urinary: Burning urination. Cystitis; last few drops burn
             and sting. Urine retention.
Women: Painful swelling of breasts or genitalia. Oedema in
             pregnancy.
Heart & Circulation: Angina. Palpitations.
Respiratory: Panting breathing. Oedema of larynx.
             Allergic asthma.
Skin: Red, sore and hot. Stinging rashes. Urticaria.
             Swellings. Boils that are red, hot and swollen.
Fever: Burning heat. Hot but thirstless.
Worse For: Heat. Touch. Pressure.
Better For: Cool.
Compare: Arsenicum, Lachesis, Sulphur.

ARNICA   ARNICA MONTANA
Common Names: Leopard's bane, Mountain tobacco
Made From: Potentised fresh plant tincture.

Mental & General
Main accident and trauma remedy. Kickstarts the healing process.
Give following any trauma mental or physical. Haemorrhage.
Bruising. Relieves shock. Helps prevent infection. Promotes healing. Over-exertion. Muscles feel sore, painful and bruised. Give
before and after operations, dental treatment, childbirth. Gunshot
wounds. Fears being touched and further injury. Says nothing is
wrong with them when clearly it is. Bed feels too hard. Coma.

Physical
Head: Injury. Meningitis following head injury. Vertigo.
Eyes: Bloodshot.
Nose: Bleeds following exertion, trauma or sneezing or
             coughing.
Women: Soreness after labour. Haemorrhage. Threatened
             miscarriage following falls, trauma, etc. Puerperal
             fever. Mastitis. Breast tumours following injury.
Heart & Circulation: Sudden pains in heart. Angina, worse
             exertion. Palpitations. Assists absorption of blood
             clots.
Skin: Painful acne. Crops of small boils.
Fever: Septic fever; especially following trauma.
Worse For: Injuries. Bruises. Shock. Touch.
Compare: Aconite, Hypericum, Rhus tox, Ruta, Symphytum.

ARSENICUM ARSENICUM ALBUM

Common Name: Metallic arsenic
Made From: Trituration and solution of arsenic trioxide.

Mental & General

A profoundly acting remedy with marked mental and physical symptoms. The remedy is for people who are critical, fastidious, demanding and anxious. It is suitable for people who have suffered great loss and are left feeling intensely anxious, fearful and agitated. Great anguish. Fears death, loss of property, disease. Restlessness. Mania. Fear of being left alone. Irritable. Wake at 1am feeling very anxious. Physical symptoms include thin, acrid and scanty secretions. Burning pains. Unusually, burning pains are relieved by warmth. Sudden great weakness. Putrid states with offensive odour. Malignancy. Allergic reactions.

Physical

Eyes: Burning tears. Conjunctivitis. Eyelids red, swollen, ulcerated.

Nose: Thin, watery, burning discharge. Cold sores in nose. Sneezing.

Digestion: Vomiting and purging. Intense thirst for sips of water. Gastritis. Burning, foul diarrhoea. Gastroenteritis (main remedy). Dysentery. Cholera. Sore, itching or burning anus. Peritonitis.

Urinary: Burning, scanty urine. Retention of urine. Albuminaria.

Respiratory: Shortness of breath. Asthma; wakes around midnight, with anxiety, relieved by sitting up in bed. Allergic asthma. Breathlessness. Bloody expectoration.

Heart & Circulation: Weak heart. Palpitations. Angina.

Extremities: Neuralgia. Cramps in calves. Paralysis with contraction of limbs. Sciatica relieved by warmth.

Skin: Looks seared. Urticaria. Rough, scaly, burning rashes. Allergic skin reactions that itch and burn. Eczema. Ulcers; with burning pains. Gangrene. Boils and carbuncles.

Fever: Chills alternating with heat. Hectic fever. Malaria. Septic fever.

Worse For: Exact periodicity. Midnight or 1am. Cold. Bad food. Drinking liquids. Exertion.

Better For: Hot applications. Hot food or drink. Lying with head propped up. Company.

Compare: Carbo veg, Lachesis, Phosphorus, Pulsatilla, Sulphur.

BELLADONNA ATROPA BELLADONNA

Common Name: Deadly Nightshade
Made From: Potentised tincture of whole plant when
           beginning to flower.

Mental & General

A most important remedy for fevers and inflammations. This is a remedy of extremes; the fever is very high, the person is very hot. Childhood illnesses. Sudden, violent fevers with burning heat and bright redness. Redness in streaks. Inflammation: give for the early, inflammatory stage of any infection, eg. boil, abscess, wound, etc. Fulness and congestion. Severe neuralgic or throbbing pain. Dryness. Nervous system affected: jerks and twitchings. Convulsions. Sunstroke. Wild delirium. Violent during fever. Angry. Restless. Give for any fever even when in doubt about cause. Give for meningitis symptoms while awaiting emergency services/medical treatment.

Physical

Head: Congestion. Throbbing or hammering headache.
              Rolls head. From sunstroke.
Eyes: Dilated pupils. Staring eyes. Conjunctivitis.
              Intense photophobia.
Face: Fiery, red face. Neuralgia.
Throat: Hot and dry. Tonsillitis.
Women: Severe period pains with profuse menses. Masititis;
              breasts heavy, hard and red with throbbing pains.
Respiratory: Short, dry or barking cough.
Skin: Inflammatory stage of any infection.
              Redness. Dry and hot.
Fever: High fever. Head hot with cold extremities.
Worse For: Heat of sun. Drafts. Checked sweat. Hair cut.
Compare: Aconite, Hepar sulph, Hyocyamus, Stramonium.

BRYONIA
BRYONIA ALBA

Common Name: White Bryony, Wild Hops
Made From: Potentised tincture of root
gathered before flowering.

Mental & General
Affects mucous membranes. Symptoms of dryness. Heavy, bursting or stitching pains. Every symptom is worse for movement. The person will hold the head or chest or other painful part to stop it moving. An important remedy for dry coughs, headaches, bowel problems, flus and muscular problems. The person is very irritable and wants to be left alone. Wants to go home. A worrier. Worries about business. Feels dull.

Physical
Head:	Bursting, heavy or splitting headache, mainly above the eyes. Headache worse when constipated. Vertigo and dizziness, worse on rising up. Sensitive scalp.
Face:	Dusky, bloated. Dry lips.
Throat:	Dry. Feels scraped or swollen.
Stomach:	Very thirsty. Desires cold water. Heaviness in stomach. Vomits solid food.
Abdomen & Stools:	Liver sore and swollen. Jaundice. Abdomen tender. Appendicitis, peritonitis. Constipation: stools large, dry and hard. Diarrhoea: gushing on rising in the morning, or from cold drinks.
Women:	Mastitis: breasts hard, hot and painful.
Respiratory:	Descending colds. Cough: dry, hard and very painful. Holds chest when coughing. Bronchitis, asthma, pneumonia, pleurisy. Sharp stitching pain in chest. Cough worse at night, eating, coming into a warm room. Cough relieved by sitting up.
Back:	Stiff neck and back. Pain worse motion.
Extremities:	Joints red, swollen and hot. Sciatica. Sprains, strains, rheumatism all worse movement.
Fever:	Painful continued fevers. Develops slowly. Dry heat.
Worse For:	Any movement, stooping, coughing, exertion, deep breathing. Becoming heated, hot weather.
Better For:	Pressure; lying on or holding painful part. Cool. Open air.
Compare:	Natrum mur, Rhus tox.

CAMPHOR   CAMPHORA

Common Name: Camphor
Made From: Potentised solution of the gum obtained from
           Laurus camphora

Mental & General

Most often used for the stage of dry collapse, with little vomiting
or purging, in cholera. Symptoms of sudden collapse and weakness. Tetanic spasms and convulsions. Patient becomes icy cold but
does not want to be covered. Loss of senses. Loss of consciousness.

Physical

Face:	Cold sweat. Lockjaw. Grimaces.
Abdomen & Stools:	Asiatic cholera. Rice water stools.
Fever:	Shaking chill. Alternation of heat and chill. Icy cold. Rapid prostration.
Worse For:	Cold.
Better For:	Free secretions.
Compare:	Carbo veg, Cuprum, Opium.

CANTHARIS   CANTHARIS VESICATORIA

Common Name: Spanish Fly
Made From: Potentised tincture of the insect.

Mental & General

Acts especially on the urinary and sexual organs. Most commonly
used for cystitis. A remedy of great irritation and inflammation.
Also useful for the pain of burns and scalds. The person feels very
angry and agitated.

Physical

Throat:	Scalding or burning pain. Painful constriction. Blisters.
Urinary:	Pain on urination is scalding, burning or cutting. Intolerable urging to urinate. Bloody urine. Cystitis, nephritis, renal colic. Kidney region sensitive.
Men:	Painful swelling of genitals.
Women:	Assists expulsion of dead foetus or placenta. Intense itching of genital area.
Skin:	Vesicular eruptions. Eruptions burn and itch, turn black. Painful burns and scalds. Radiation burns. Blistering caused by chemical exposure.
Worse For:	Urination. Cold drinks. Sexual excitement.
Compare:	Apis, Arsenicum, Mercurius.

CARBO VEG   CARBO VEGETABILIS
Common Name: Vegetable Charcoal
Made From: Potentised trituration of wood charcoal.

Mental & General
A key life-saver remedy for severe weakness. Weakness may be
due to loss of vital fluids, eg. blood, disease or effects of poisoning. It is known as the 'corpse reviver' as it may revive those who
look close to death. Give to those nearly drowned. Lack of reaction to other treatments or remedies. Collapse. It may revive new
born infants when close to death, 'blue babies'. Symptoms of
decay, stagnation and putrefaction. Blueness and poor circulation. Flatulence. Air hunger. Well suited to elderly people. Yellow
fever. Mentally they will appear irritable, slow and anxious.

Physical
Face: Pinched, looks aged. Pale, bluish or dusky.
Stomach: Nausea. Rancid, loud burping. Heaviness and
            fullness after eating. Gastralgia, dyspepsia, ulcers.
            Vomits blood.
Abdomen & Stools: Great flatulence. Any food causes discom-
            fort. Burning in rectum. Colic. Jaundice.
Respiratory: Craves air. Tormenting cough. Whooping cough
            or asthma with bluish face. Burning in larynx or
            chest. Laboured breathing.
Skin: Blue, cold. Ulcers: bleeding, burning, gangrenous.
Fever: Extremities cold. Internal burning heat.
Worse For: Rich food. Excess. Warmth. Loss of vital fluids.
Better For: Burping. Cool air or fanning.
Compare: Ant tart, Arsenicum, China.

CAUSTICUM CAUSTICUM

Common Name: Potassium hydrate, caustic potash
Made From: Potentised tincture obtained by distilling a mixture
of lime and potassium sulphate solution.

Mental & General

An important remedy for the nerves and muscles. Symptoms
include weakness, paralysis, trembling and jerking. Pains are sore,
raw and burning. Bladder weakness. Relieves the pain and promotes healing of deep burns, radiation burns. May be used to treat
old burns and scars. Mentally they are oversensitive and overly anxious about others. Suffers long after loss or bereavement. Anxious.
Pessimistic. Absent minded.

Physical

Face: Neuralgia. Paralysis; Bell's palsy.
Respiratory: Hoarseness that is worse after speaking or singing.
             Laryngitis. Cough hard, dry, from tickling in
             throat. Cough relieved by sips of water. Cannot
             cough deep enough; expectoration slips back
             again. Chest sore and tight.
Extremities: Trembling of hands. Paralysis. Numbness. Cramps
             in calves, feet and toes.
Skin: Cracked and sore. Ulcers.
             Scars slow to heal; reopen.
             Deep burns and their effects.
Worse For: Dry, cold air. Wind. Drafts. Evening.
Compare: Phosphorus, Rhus tox.

CHAMOMILLA   MATRICARIA CHAMOMILLA

Common Name: Chamomile, German Chamomile
Made From: Potentised tincture of whole fresh plant.

Mental & General

All pain is felt intensely and with great oversensitivity. Intolerable pain. Irritable, bad tempered, restless and emotional patient. A useful remedy for infants and during pregnancy. Teething troubles. They are angry, demanding, very contrary and quarrelsome. Child wants to be carried all the time. Hates being talked to, touched or looked at.

Physical

Ears:	Earache.
Face:	Redness of one cheek. Neuralgia.
Mouth:	Toothache; worse after warm drinks, during pregnancy, of teething children.
Abdomen & Stools:	Colic with cutting pains, worse at night. Stools are sour, slimy, yellow or green, smells like rotten eggs. Diarrhoea when teething.
Women:	Period pains with clotted, dark blood. Labour pains intolerable. After pains of labour.
Respiratory:	Dry, tickling or rattling cough in children. Asthma worse after anger.
Fever:	Chills and heat alternating. Coldness of one part with heat of another.
Worse For:	Anger. Night. Teething. Coffee. Drugs. Getting cold.
Better For:	Being carried (children). Sweating.
Compare:	Belladonna, Nux vomica, Staphysagria.

CHINA CHINCHONA OFFICINALIS

Common Name: Peruvian bark
Made From: Potentised tincture of the dried bark.

Mental & General

Affects the blood. Debility due to profuse and exhausting discharges. Haemorrhages. Anaemia. Collapse. Intermittent fever; malaria. Used as a prophylactic against malaria. Given after blood loss can help stimulate haemoglobin production and prevent need for transfusion. Hepatitis. People needing this remedy are oversensitive, nervous and easily upset. Or they may appear surprisingly indifferent. Day dreaming.

Physical

Head: Bursting, throbbing headache. Vertigo.
Ears: Tinnitus.
Stomach: Bitter or sour burping. Anorexia; feels full all the
            time, aversion to food. Loud belching; does not
            bring relief.
Abdomen & Stools: Flatulence. Bloating. Colic. Post-operative
            gas pains. Liver disease. Gall stone colic. Jaundice.
            Stools; undigested food, bloody, dark, foul, watery,
            painless. Diarrhoea worse after eating, becomes
            chronic.
Respiratory: Bloody expectoration. Asthma worse damp
            weather or with depletion. Painful, sore chest.
Fever: Intermittent fever; stages of chill, heat and sweat.
            Hot face with cold hands. Drenching sweats; worse
            night, motion. Tropical fevers. Septic fevers.
Worse For: Vital losses. Touch. Jarring. Noise. Periodically.
            Cold. Wind. Draughts. Fruit. Eating. Milk.
            Bad food. Tea.
Better For: Hard pressure.
Compare: Arsenicum, Carbo veg.

COLOCYNTH
COLOCYNTHUS

Common Name: Bitter Apple
Made From: Potentised tincture of pulp of fruit

Mental & General
This is primarily a remedy for colic. There are sudden, violent, cutting, gripping pains in the digestive system. Also neuralgia, especially of the face. The symptoms may come on after being very angry or worked up about something. Or the pain may cause feelings of anger. Colic in children, especially when relieved by bending over or doubling up.

Physical
Face: Neuralgia. Face becomes distorted.
Stomach: Pain. Vomits from pain.
Abdomen & Stools: Severe colicky pains. Pains come in waves. Person presses on stomach to relieve pain, or bends double, because pains are relieved by pressure. Pains aggravated by any food or drink. Stools are frothy, watery or yellow. Painful flatulence. Acute or chronic diarrhoea. Dysentery. Infantile colic.
Worse For: Being angry. Night.
Better For: Hard pressure. Heat. Rest. Doubling up.

CROTALUS
CROTALUS HORRIDUS

Common Name: Rattle-snake
Made From: Potentised trituration of milk sugar saturated with venom.

Mental & General
An important remedy for putrid, malignant conditions. Deathly sickness with decomposition, trembling and prostration. Slow, oozing haemorrhages. Blood may ooze out of every orifice. Septic, gangrenous states. Septicaemia. Radiation exposure. Delirium. Dementia. Melancholy. Horrible dreams.

Physical
Face: Death like pallor. Yellow. Lips swollen.
Mouth: Mouldy breath. Swollen tongue.
            Constriction of tongue and throat.
Stomach: Vomiting; bilious, of blood, cannot retain anything. Vomiting, purging and urination simultaneously.

Abdomen & Stools: Swollen abdomen. Peritonitis.
Haemorrhage from anus. Malignant jaundice.
Icy coldness. Stools black.
Women: Puerperal fever.
Skin: Jaundiced. Haemorrhages. Septic boils, carbuncles,
            abscesses. Oedema around affected part. Gangrene.
Fever: Malignant fevers. Yellow fever. Meningitis. Sweat
            cold or bloody.
Worse For: Lying on right side. Sleep. Spring.
Compare: Lachesis, Pyrogen.

FERRUM PHOS   FERRUM PHOSPHORICUM ALBUM
Common Name: White phosphate of iron
Made From: Trituration obtained after mixing sodium phos-
           phate and iron sulphate.

Mental & General
The oxygen carrying tissue salt which affects the blood and circulation. Used for local congestion, inflammation, haemorrhages
and anaemia. Helpful in the first stage of any acute illness where
there is inflammation and fever. Nosebleeds. It can be used to
stem the flow of blood from cuts, and help to prevent infection,
by crushing a few pills and sprinkling the powder onto the
injured part.

Physical
Head: Throbbing headache. Headache with earache.
            Sunstroke.
Ears: Acute earache. Deafness with a cold.
Nose: Stems flow of nosebleed.
Throat: First stage of sore throat. Hoarseness. Laryngitis.
Abdomen & Stools: Bloody diarrhoea. Summer diarrhoea.
            Dysentery with fever.
Respiratory: Laryngitis. Tickling cough. Blood streaked expecto-
            ration. Congestion of lung. Pleurisy. Pneumonia.
Heart & Circulation: Palpitations. Rapid pulse. Strengthens
            blood vessel walls. Anaemia.
Fever: First stages of colds or flu. Chill. Continued, infec-
            tious fevers. Measles. Rheumatic.
Worse For: Night. Checked sweat. Cold. Motion.
Compare: Aconite, Belladonna, Gelsemium.

GELSEMIUM   GELSEMIUM SEMPERVIRENS
Common Name: Yellow jasmine
Made From: Potentised tincture obtained from bark of the root.

Mental & General
Gelsemium acts mainly on muscles, motor nerves and mucous membranes. The classic flu remedy. Functional paralysis or twitchings. Trembling from weakness or trembling from fright. Muscles refuse to obey the will. Polio. Anticipatory anxiety. Great fear of losing control. Fear and dread before an ordeal, eg. travelling, exams, public speaking. Stage fright. Feels cannot cope and gives up. Drowsy and confused.

Physical

Head:	Vertigo. Dull heavy headache.
Eyes:	Heavy, drooping eyelids. Visual disturbance with headache. Eyes aching.
Nose:	Thin, watery discharge. Sneezing.
Face:	Dusky, red, congested appearance. Paralysis.
Throat:	Swallowing difficult. Sore.
Respiratory:	Hoarseness. Dry cough.
Extremities:	Trembling.
Fever:	Chill with aching. Heat alternating with chills. Chill up and down spine. Thirst absent. Flu. Typhoid.
Worse For:	Dread, before an ordeal. Strong emotions. Humid weather. Heat of sun.
Better For:	Urination. Sweating. Alcoholic drinks.

HEPAR SULPH   HEPAR SULPHURIS CALCAREUM
Common Name: Sulphide of calcium.
Made From: The white inside of an oyster shell is burned
together with flowers of sulphur and then triturated.

Mental & General
An important remedy where there is suppuration, abscesses, boils and infections. The main remedy to think of for the pussy stage of an abscess, wound, boil, etc. Copious thick pus. The infected area is very painful and they feel it must not be touched. Every pain is a torment. The patient becomes oversensitive, chilly and touchy mentally and physically. Sharp, stitching pains. Violent impulses and a nasty temperament. Hasty.

70

Physical

Eyes:	Ulcers.
Ears:	Darting pain. Mastoiditis.
Mouth:	Main remedy for dental abscess. Ulcers. Offensive breath.
Throat:	Swelling of tonsils and glands. Hawks mucus. Stitching pain extends to ear when swallowing.
Respiratory:	Choking, tickling cough. Hoarseness. Weakness in chest. Rattling in chest. Thick, yellow expectoration. Bronchitis. Asthma.
Skin:	Eruptions in folds of skin. Painful boils, ulcers or abscess. Chapped, cracked skin. Painful cold sores. Impetigo.
Fever:	Septic fevers. Profuse sweat. Night sweats.
Worse For:	Cold; air, wind, drafts. Touch.
Better For:	Warm covering.

HYPERICUM   HYPERICUM PERFORATUM

Common Name: St John's Wort
Made From: Potentised tincture of whole fresh plant.

General

An important remedy for injury to parts rich in nerves, ie. fingers, toes, spine. Lacerated wounds. Painful injuries. Neuralgia. Pain in old injuries. Acts as an antiseptic for any suppurating or slow to heal wounds. Prophylactic for tetanus (give Ledum first then follow with Hypericum especially if there is any sign of infection).

Physical

Neck&Back:	After-effects of injury to spine. Spinal concussion. Pain in spine or coccyx. Back pain after childbirth.
Extremities:	Painful injuries. Injury to nail bed. Sciatica. Neuralgia in stump after loss of limb.
Skin:	Wounds; lacerated, gaping, deep punctured. Gunshot wounds. Painful scars. Insect bites become infected. Give following any sign of infection developing.
Worse For:	Injury. Jar. Motion. Concussion. Shock. Insect bites.
Compare:	Arnica, Ledum, Rhus tox, Ruta.

71

IGNATIA

IGNATIA AMARA

Common Name: St Ignatius' Bean
Made From: Potentised tincture obtained from the seeds.

Mental & General

One of the most important remedies for treating acute mental and emotional trauma, shock and distress. Symptoms that come on following the death of a loved one, bad news, disappointment, etc. Grief with sighing. The person is unable to express their grief appropriately. Symptoms are erratic and contradictory. Nervous system affects including spasms, twitching, shuddering, rigidity and trembling. Hysteria. Effects of bereavement, loss and grief. Emotional shock. Person becomes oversensitive and nervous, or may become silent and unable to cry or grieve. Unhappy love affairs. Inappropriate laughter. Hasty. Changeable. Hysterical.

Physical

Head:	Pain in small spot; as if a nail driven in. Vertigo.
Throat:	Globus hystericus. Pain as of a lump. Choking.
Stomach:	Empty sinking feeling. Nausea. Hiccoughs.
Abdomen:	Shooting pain in rectum. Colic.
Extremities:	Trembling, jerking and twitching. Cramps.
Worse For:	Emotional shock, grief, worry. Touch. Coffee. Cigarette smoke.
Compare:	Aconite, Natrum mur, Nux vomica, Pulsatilla, Staphysagria.

IPECAC CEPHAELIS IPECACUANHA

Common Name: Ipecacuanha
Made From: Potentised tincture obtained from dried root.

General
An important remedy in the treatment of nausea and haemorrhages. Also respiratory complaints. Constant nausea with any
complaint. First remedy for haemorrhages that are bright red and
gushing.

Physical
Stomach: Constant horrid nausea, not relieved by vomiting.
            Nausea with a clean tongue. Morning sickness of
            pregnancy. Sinking feeling in stomach. Vomits
            blood or mucus.
Abdomen & Stools: Cutting pain around navel. Bloody,
            mucussy or slimy diarrhoea. Dysentery.
Women: Bright red, gushing uterine haemorrhage. Steady
            flow of bright red blood. Haemorrhage following
            miscarriage, childbirth or of placenta praevia.
Respiratory: Suffocative cough; comes in paroxysms, ends with
            retching and vomiting. Asthma. Whooping cough.
            Gasps for breath. During cough child stiffens out.
            Loose rattling in chest without expectoration.
            Bronchitis. Broncho-pneumonia.
Fever: Nausea with fever. Gastric flu.
Worse For: Warmth. Damp. Overeating or rich foods.
            Vomiting.
Compare: Nux vomica, Phosphorus.

LACHESIS TRIGONOCEPHALUS LACHESIS

Common Name: Bushmaster or Surukuku Snake.
Made From: Potentised snake venom in alcohol.

Mental & Physical

An important remedy for septic conditions. Affects the blood and circulation. Affected parts look blue or purple. Most symptoms are left sided. Flushes of heat. Feeling of a lump. The person feels much worse in the sun and in the morning after sleep. Symptoms are very painful. Delusions. Talkative. The person becomes jealous and suspicious.

Physical

Throat:	Feeling of a lump. Pains extend to the ear on swallowing. Cannot bear anything tight around neck. Swollen tonsils. Foul, thick mucus. Diphtheria.
Abdomen & Stool:	Inflamed liver. Septic gall bladder. Appendicitis. Abdomen hot and sensitive. Foul haemorrhage from bowels. Urging and pain in rectum.
Women:	Menses are dark and offensive. Breast painful, inflamed, blue. Hot flushes of menopause.
Respiratory:	Sensation of suffocation especially on going to sleep. Shortness of breath. Fluid on lung. Bloody or frothy expectoration.
Circulation:	Palpitations. Weak pulse. Cyanosis.
Skin:	Mottled, bluish or purple discoloration. Ulcers. Bed sores. Copious bleeding from small wounds. Gunshot wounds. Gangrene.
Fever:	Flushes of heat. Sweat; bloody, yellow, staining. Cold extremities.
Worse For:	Sleep. On waking. Morning. Spring. Heat of sun. Swallowing. Touch. Pressure of clothes. Checked discharges. Hot drinks. Alcohol. Before menses. Menopause.
Better For:	Cool. Open air. Discharges. Cold drinks. Hard pressure.
Compare:	Lycopodium, Sepia.

LEDUM   LEDUM PALUSTRE
Common Name: Marsh Tea, Marsh Cistus, Wild Rosemary.
Made From: Tincture of whole fresh plant collected when flowering.

General
Affected parts become puffy, swollen and purplish. Give immediately after a puncture wound to prevent tetanus. Insect and
animal bites and stings. First remedy for wasp or hornet stings.
Bruising.

Physical
Eyes:	Injury – black eye. Haemorrhage.
Extremities:	Pains in ball of foot, heel or toe.
	Ankles sprain easily. Tendonitis.
Skin:	Puncture wounds. Twitching around wound.
	Puffy swelling.
Worse For:	Injury. Moving affected part.
Better For:	Cool bathing of affected part.
Compare:	Arnica, Hypericum, Rhus tox.

MERCURIUS, MERC SOL   MERCURIUS SOLUBILIS
Common Name: Mercury, Quicksilver
Made From: Soluble black oxide of mercury precipitated from a
           solution in nitric acid by using caustic ammonia
           then potentised.

Mental & General
Affects the lymphatic glands, and especially salivary glands. Glands
become swollen and discharge. The two key themes are offen-
siveness of mind and body and an increase in secretions. All secretions are increased and become offensive. Suppurations. Ulcers.
Weakness and exhaustion. Muscles are affected with tremblings,
twitchings and paralysis or disordered movements. An important
remedy for dysentery. Mercurius is for those who are hasty, lack
stability and tend to have unpleasant habits. Hurried, stammer-
ing and nervous. Violent or disgusting impulses. Suicidal thoughts.
Loss of memory or will power.

Physical
Head:	Vertigo. Headache with toothache or earache.
	Meningitis; child turns head from side to side.
	Oily sweat.
Face:	Swollen glands. Mumps. Looks yellow.
	Eyelids swollen.

Ears: Pains extend to ear from teeth or throat. Thick, yellow discharge. Boils.

Nose: Much sneezing. Colds travel up to eyes. Sinusitis.

Mouth: Breath horribly offensive. Bleeding, swollen gums. Gumboils. Mouth ulcers or thrush. Increased salivation; flows during sleep. Indented, flabby tongue. Metallic taste in mouth.

Throat: Sore, burning or raw throat. Swollen tonsils. Ulcerated tonsils. Pain into ears on swallowing. Hawks mucus.

Abdomen & Stools: Liver enlarged and sore. Jaundice. Stools; bloody, slimy, offensive. Never get done feeling with stool; constant urging. Swelling of inguinal glands. Appendicitis. Dysentery.

Urination: Increased urine. Burning after urination.

Skin: Easy perspiration. Oily perspiration. Moist eruptions. Ulcers; bleeding, spreading, irregular. Itching with jaundice.

Fever: Easily overheated then chilled. Measles. Profuse sweating without relief. Fever and sweating worse at night.

Worse For: Night. Sweating. Heat. Cold. Changing weather.

Better For: Moderate temperature.

Compare: Belladonna, Hepar sulph, Silica.

NATRUM MUR — NATRUM MURIATICUM
Common Name: Sodium chloride, Common salt
Made From: Potentised trituration of mineral salt.

Mental & Physical
People needing this remedy tend to be serious and reserved and dislike fuss and attention. They usually crave salt. They tend to be easily offended and can become resentful and depressed. They may feel tearful but have difficulty in expressing emotion, or may go off by themselves to cry. Physically they tend to have symptoms of dryness, or water retention and oedema. An important remedy in the treatment of malaria, especially if prolonged or never fully recovered from. Depression and sadness especially following disappointment, misfortune, grief, etc. Hates consolation and fuss. Remembers any slight or offence against them. Becomes resentful and desires revenge. Fears and nightmares, especially of robbers. Talks in sleep. Can become averse to company. Loss of speech through grief.

Physical

Head: Vertigo as if falling. Headaches; hammering, bursting, over eyes, worse on waking up. Disturbed vision with headache. Migraine. Alopecia.

Eyes: Watering.

Nose: Watery discharge; dripping. Discharge and dryness alternating. Loss of smell and taste.

Face: Cold sores. Crack in middle of lower lip. Dry lips.

Stomach: Craves salt. Thirsty. Heartburn.

Abdomen & Stools: Tendency to constipation: with dry, hard, crumbling stools.

Women: Painful intercourse with dryness and burning. Menses absent or too profuse. Herpes around genitals.

Skin: Herpetic eruptions. Hives. Eruptions around margins of hair.

Fever: Coldness of extremities. Intermittent fever. Fever returns with exact periodicity. Malaria.

Worse For: Mornings. Alternate days. Heat of sun. Sympathy. Mental exertion.

Better For: Open air. Sweating.

Compare: Ignatia, Pulsatilla, Sepia.

NATRUM SULPH NATRUM SULPHURICUM

Common Name: Glauber's Salt

Made From: Trituration and solution of sodium sulphate.

Mental & General

A remedy for complaints caused by living in damp houses, basements, etc. An important liver remedy: jaundice, hepatitis. All discharges are yellow and the skin is yellowish. Chronic asthma. Give this remedy after Arnica following head injury. Mental problems that follow head injury. Suicidal impulses.

Physical

Head: Reduces inflammation following head injury. Epilepsy following head injury.

Abdomen & Stools: Liver area sore. Painful flatulence. Diarrhoea - rumbling and gurgling in the bowels and then sudden spluttering, noisy stools. Diarrhoea first thing in the morning.

Respiratory: Asthma follows every cold. Asthma worse after exertion or in damp weather.

Worse For: Damp - weather, rooms. Injury.

NUX VOMICA STRYCHNOS NUX VOMICA
Common Name: Poison Nut
Made From: Potentised tincture of seeds.

Mental & General
The main actions are on the nervous system and the digestion. There are spasms, twitching and impaired or reversed peristalsis. It is for those who are critical, exacting, ambitious and forceful. They become hypersensitive and irritable. Nausea. An important remedy for the ill effects of drugs or alcohol: hangover. Angry, impatient and irritable. Can not bear pain. Violent impulses. Hypochondriasis. Insomnia: wakes up too early and cannot go back to sleep.

Physical
Nose:	Violent sneezing. Discharge in day, dries up at night. Acute sense of smell.
Stomach:	Hiccups. Terrible nausea that is relieved by vomiting. Violent vomiting. Gastralgia. Indigestion worse after rich or spicy food, which is craved. Water brash. Pain in stomach after injury. Nausea of radiation exposure.
Abdomen & Stools:	Sore abdomen. Gall stone colic. Hepatitis with jaundice. Umbilical hernia. Colic. Constipation with fitful urging for stool; or part of stool remains after straining. Rectal spasm. Itching haemorrhoids. Dysentery; feels better immediately after stool. Diarrhoea causes prolapse of rectum. Cannot bear tight clothes.
Urination:	Suppressed urination. Paralysis of bladder. Renal colic.
Women:	Severe cramping menstrual pains. Menses profuse and early.
Respiratory:	Violent spasmodic cough. Cough causes headache. Asthma.
Fever:	Easily chilled. Hot to the touch but feels chilled.
Worse For:	Rich foods. Excess alcohol. Tight clothing. Early morning. Cold.
Better For:	Free discharges; after vomiting, or stool.
Compare:	Arsenicum, Phosphorus, Sulphur.

OPIUM   PAPAVER SOMNIFERUM
Common Name: Opium poppy
Made From: Potentised tincture of opium.

Mental & General
Symptoms are due to suppression or inactivity of nerves and senses. An important remedy for the after effects of a severe trauma or shock or the sight of an accident. The fear of the fright remains. Lack of reaction. Paralysis especially of brain or bowels. Drowsiness. Loss of consciousness. Drowsy and stupor. They may withdraw into their own inner world. They lose judgement and behave inappropriately or rashly, hence fearless. Become unaffected by pain or indifferent emotionally. Fears and nightmares after a fright. Effects of fright remain for a prolonged time.

Physical
Abdomen & Stools: Bowels obstructed or paralysed. Loss of bowel function following an operation or injury. Obstinate constipation. Stools hard, dark, like balls. Colic.
Urination: Paralytic bladder after operation or injury. Retention of urine.
Women: Threatened miscarriage from fright.
Respiratory: Sighing, rattling or uneven breathing.
Heart & Circulation: Slow full pulse. Palpitations following fright.
Extremities: Trembling limbs. Paralysis after fright. Numbness.
Skin: Itching all over.
Fever: Hot sweat. Drowsy.
Worse For: Fear or trauma. Alcohol. Suppressed discharges. Sleep. Heat.
Compare: Aconite, Ignatia, Phos ac.

PHOS AC   PHOSPHORICUM ACIDUM
Common Name: Phosphoric acid
Made From: Potentised solution of the acid.

Mental & General
Affects mainly the mind and the nervous system. It covers many symptoms of weakness, debility and exhaustion. The after effects of struggling with adversity or traumatic experiences. The person appears to 'give up' and become exhausted. Slow reactions. Indifference and apathy. Far away look. Slow grasp of things. Poor memory and concentration. Hopelessness. Dread of the future. Home sick. Sleepy in the day but insomnia at night.

Physical
Head: Crushing, heavy headache. Vertigo: as if floating. Alopecia.

Face: Eyes look sunken, with dark or blue rings around them.

Abdomen & Stools: Stools; watery, or undigested food. Diarrhoea; watery, gushing, but painless. Involuntary stools.

Women: Exhaustion due to prolonged breastfeeding.

Infants: Cannot keep any milk down.

Back: Paralytic weakness of spine. Burning pain along spine.

Extremities: Pins and needles. Cramps. Numbness.

Fever: Profuse sweat during fever. Prolonged fever with no other symptoms.

Worse For: Loss of vital fluids. Exhaustion. Emotions; grief, fright. Cold.

Better For: Warmth.

Compare: Aconite, China, Ignatia, Opium.

PHOSPHORUS   PHOSPHORUS
Common Name: Phosphorus
Made From: Potentised trituration of red phosphorus.

Mental & General
Great tendency to haemorrhage. Illnesses which gradually worsen, become debilitating and destructive. Burning pains. An important remedy for restless, nervous, fearful people. And those who

are outgoing, desire company and like to be comforted. Symptoms especially of the nervous system, lungs, stomach, blood vessels or bones. Fearful; of being alone, dark, ghosts, imaginings, thunderstorms, the future, disease. Nervous and 'jumpy'. Liveliness followed by exhaustion. Excitable, alternating with apathy and indifference. Delusions of grandeur. Amorous. Excitement followed by flushes of heat. Enjoys a short sleep in the day, wakeful at night. Important remedy for the after effects of radiation exposure: nausea, haemorrhage, burns.

Physical

Nose: Fan like motion of nostrils. Nose colds descend to the chest. Nosebleeds.

Stomach: Craves food or drinks (especially cold) which are vomited soon after eating or drinking. Frequent vomiting. Drinks cold water that is vomited as soon as it warms in the stomach.
Ravenous hunger; empty feeling in stomach.
Nausea following general anaesthetic.
Vomits blood. Burning in stomach. Water brash.

Abdomen & Stools: Stools: thin, foul, watery, gushing, with blood. Exhausting diarrhoea. Dysentery. Anal haemorrhage. Burning in rectum. Acute hepatitis. Malignant jaundice. Atrophy of liver.

Women: Uterine haemorrhage: sudden, during childbirth.

Respiratory: Tightness of chest. Raw, sore larynx with a husky voice. Bronchitis. Tickling, painful, hacking cough. Copious expectoration. Haemorrhage of lung. Pneumonia.

Extremities: Paralysis moves upwards from fingers and toes. Pins and needles. Burning pains in bones. Osteomyelitis. Cramps. Numbness, weakness and trembling of limbs. Icy coldness.

Skin: Even small wounds bleed a lot. Ulcers. Fungal infections. Easy bruising. Radiation burns.

Fever: Burning heat. Hectic fevers. Craves ice. Painless fevers.

Worse For: After excitement or strong emotions. Cold. Sexual excess. Twilight. Exhaustion.

Better For: Sleep. Rubbing. Cold food.

Compare: Arsenicum, Causticum, Ipecac (in haemorrhage), Nux vomica, Pulsatilla.

PODOPHYLLUM PODOPHYLLUM PELTATUM
Common Name: May Apple, American Mandrake
Made From: Potentised tincture obtained from root.

General
Mainly affects the liver, duodenum and rectum. An important remedy for diarrhoea and dysentery. Diarrhoea alternating with other symptoms, ie. constipation, headache. Jaundiced look.

Physical
Mouth: Offensive smell. Bitter taste.

Stomach: Constant gagging and retching. Heartburn. Infants vomit milk.

Abdomen & Stools: Liver area sore; relieved by rubbing. Sinking feeling. Gurgling noises followed by gushing diarrhoea. Painless diarrhoea. Stools: watery, white, foamy. Summer diarrhoea. Diarrhoea alternating with constipation. Rectum: sore, raw, weak, prolapsed. Involuntary stools.

Women: Tendency to prolapse: uterus and rectum. Diarrhoea during pregnancy or after childbirth.

Fever: During or alternating with diarrhoea. Profuse, offensive sweat.

Worse For: Early morning. After eating. Acidic fruit or food. Hot weather. Milk.

Better For: Rubbing. Lying on abdomen.

PULSATILLA   PULSATILLA NIGRICANS
Common Name: Pasque Flower
Made From: Potentised tincture of entire fresh plant when in
flower.

Mental & Emotional
An important remedy with a wide range of symptoms. It is suited
to people who are mild, emotional, weepy, demanding and like
sympathy. They crave company. A key indication is that the symptoms are changeable. It mainly effects the mind and emotions,
the mucous membranes and digestion. A very important remedy
for children. Main remedy for children's diseases: earaches, fevers,
mumps, measles, etc. Glandular swelling. Tearful. Becomes sad.
Weepy and irritable. Fearful of being left alone. Children become
'clingy', whine and crave fuss and attention. Also commonly indicated during pregnancy.

Physical
Eyes: Conjunctivitis from a head cold. Thick, yellow,
              bland discharges. Recurrent styes.
              Itching and burning in eyes. Weeping eyes.
Ears: Earache worse at night. Catarrhal deafness or
              earache. Earache in children. Swollen lobes.
Nose: Thick, yellow catarrh.
Mouth: Offensive breath. Bad taste. Mouth dry but with-
              out thirst. Food tastes bitter.
Stomach: Nausea. Heartburn. Thirstless. Fatty food, pork,
              and rich food disagree. Stomach feels heavy.
Abdomen & Stools: Heaviness in abdomen. Stools changeable.
              Diarrhoea from bad food, or with jaundice.
Men: Swollen testicles. Thick, yellow discharge.
Women: Periods changeable, delayed. Often indicated
              during pregnancy, childbirth and when breastfeed-
              ing. Malposition of foetus. Weak labour pains.
              Poor milk supply. Post-partum haemorrhage from
              retained placenta.
Respiratory: Shortness of breath. Cough loose in the morning,
              dry at night. Thick, slimy expectoration. Heaviness
              in chest. Cough after measles.
Fever: Chilly, yet craves fresh air. Erratic fever.
Worse For: Warmth, stuffy rooms. Evening. Lying down. Rich
              food. Puberty. Pregnancy.
Better For: Cool, fresh air. Sitting erect. After crying. Rubbing.

PYROGEN   PYROGENIUM

Common Name: Sepsin
Made From: Potentised product of decomposed chopped lean
           beef in water, allowed to stand in the sun for 2
           weeks.

Mental & General

A remedy for all septic states. Discharges are horribly foul. Blood
poisoning with red streaks on the skin. Bones ache and muscles
feel sore and bruised. Poisoning from toxic gas, dirty surgical
instruments, toxins entering the blood stream, etc. Helps clear
out the toxic effects of too many vaccinations. Puerperal fever
(after childbirth). The person feels exhausted yet restless. For
people who have never felt well since an infection. The person
suffers from delusions, especially a sense of duality. Talk to themselves. Diphtheria, typhoid, malaria, yellow fever.

Physical

Stomach: Persistent vomiting.
Abdomen & Stools: Horribly offensive stools.
Heart & Circulation: Pulse is quick and out of all proportion to
           temperature. Or the reverse. Heart failure threatens
           in septic states.
Extremities: Aching in limbs.
Skin: Red streaks. Injury becomes red and swollen. Boils.
Fever: Slowly advancing. Hectic.
            Quickly oscillating temperature.
Worse For: Cold damp. Night. Sepsis.
Better For: Warmth. Motion.
Compare: Arsenicum, Crotalus, Lachesis, Mercurius.

RADIUM   RADIUM BROMIDE

Common Name: Radium
Made From: Potentised trituration of radium bromide of
           1,800,000 radioactivity.
A remedy for the after effects of exposure to radiation. Specific
remedy for burns and ulcers due to radiation. Ulcers that take a
long time to heal. Bad effects of X-rays. Also for aching in the
bones after injury, eg. fracture. Severe bone pains.

RHUS TOX   RHUS TOXICODENDRON

Common Name: Poison Ivy, Poison Oak
Made From: Potentised tincture of fresh leaves.

Mental & General

A very important remedy for muscle pains and injuries. Give after
sprains, strains, backache from overexertion, etc. Rheumatic symptoms whether from inflammation, injury, flu, etc. Pains are sore,
bruised and stiff. The pains make the person very restless, they
keep moving restlessly and changing position to relieve the pain.
Injured parts stiffen up when kept still. Pains are also worse in
cold, damp weather or from getting wet. Also a remedy for moist,
itching skin eruptions, eg. shingles, herpes and urticaria.
Chickenpox. The person is anxious and has restless dreams.

Physical

Mouth & Throat: Sore throat. Swollen glands. Triangular red tip
on end of tongue.

Abdomen & Stools: Diarrhoea. Dysentery. Typhoid. Diarrhoea
worse after getting wet.

Extremities: Painful. Numbness. Pains follow nerve. Stiffness.
Sprains and strains.

Skin: Eruptions burn and itch. Blistering.
Moist eruptions. Eruptions on genitals or parts
covered with hair. Shingles, herpes, urticaria.
Smallpox.

Fever: Easily chilled. Restless. From getting cold and wet.
Flu. Typhoid.

Worse For: Exposure to cold and damp. Wet feet. Being
chilled. Beginning of movement. After rest. Injury.
Over exertion. Over lifting. Night.

Better For: Continued movement. Heat. Hot bath. Rubbing.

Compare: Arnica, Arsenicum, Bryonia, Ruta.

RUTA
RUTA GRAVEOLENS

Common Name: Rue
Made From: Potentised tincture of whole fresh plant.

General
A remedy for injury to fibrous tissue, especially tendons, ligaments and cartilage. Useful following any injury to elbows or knees. The main remedy for bruises to the bone, which are often very painful. Pains are sore, bruised and aching. Combines well with Rhus tox.

Physical
Neck&Back: Whiplash. Bruised feeling in back.
Extremities: Sore, bruised pains. Tendonitis.
              Legs and knees feel weak. Contractions.
Worse For: Injury. Over exertion. Sprains & strains. Cold.

SECALE
SECALE CORNUTUM

Common Name: Spurred Rye, ergot of Rye
Made From: Potentised tincture of the fresh spurs.

General
A remedy for decomposition and haemorrhage. Discharges become dark, thin and disgusting. Infected parts become very painful with burning, tingling, crawling pains. Skin infections, ulcers. Main remedy for anthrax of the skin.

Physical
Women: Uterine haemorrhage with dark, offensive dis-
            charge: after childbirth or miscarriage.
Extremities: Cramps and twitchings.
Skin: Boils, ulcers. Green pus. Foul discharges.
Fever: Internal heat yet feels cold to touch.
Worse For: Warmth. Being covered. Pregnancy.
Better For: Cool bathing. Uncovering. Stretching.

SEPIA   SEPIA OFFICINALIS

Common Name: Cuttle fish
Made From: Potentised trituration of liquid
            contained in the ink-bag.

Mental & General

The main use for Sepia is for women who have become exhausted
and dragged down by pregnancy, childbirth and overwork. It will
relieve many symptoms that come on or get worse during pregnancy, eg. morning sickness, constipation, varicose veins, piles,
backache. Mentally people needing it become anxious, angry,
touchy, irritable and easily offended. They can become indifferent and even hateful to their loved ones.

Physical

Stomach: Nausea at thought or smell of food.
             Morning sickness of pregnancy.
Abdomen & Stool: Liver region sore and painful.
             Constipation for days. Piles.
             Diarrhoea with exhaustion.
Women: Weak, dragging down sensation in uterus. Uterine
             prolapse following childbirth. Threatened miscar-
             riage especially 5th-7th months.
Worse For: Cold, pregnancy, miscarriage.
Better For: Violent motion (eg. dancing, aerobic exercise).

SILICA
SILICEA TERRA

Common Name: Flint
Made From: Potentised trituration of pure, precipitated silica.

Mental & General
The person needing this remedy lacks stamina and 'grit' mentally and physically. Symptoms tend to develop slowly and are hard to turn around, they get stuck. It affects the glands, bones, nerves and nutrition. A useful remedy for many inflammations and infections that stubbornly refuse to heal. Suppurative processes eg. abscesses, fistula. Also give for any foreign body that refuses to come out, e.g. splinters. For abscesses, boils, etc. give Hepar sulph first when the pus is gathering, and then Silica to complete the healing process.

Physical
Ears: Chronic ear infections. Perforated drum.
                Mastoiditis.
Mouth: Gum abscess.
Abdomen & Stools: Constipation. Stool when partly expelled
                recedes again. Anal fistula. Chronic diarrhoea.
Extremities: Foul foot sweat.
Skin: Unhealthy. Every small injury gets infected.
                Stubborn splinters.
Worse For: Cold. Pressure.
Better For: Warmth.
Compare: Hepar sulph.

STAPHYSAGRIA
DELPHINIUM STAPHYSAGRIA

Common Name: Stavesacre
Made From: Potentised tincture of the seeds.

Mental & General
An important remedy for the victim of any awful situation. The victim responds by being passive and yielding and allows help to pass them by. They cannot make demands or express anger. They are overwhelmed by timidity. A key remedy for violation: rape, assault, mugging, etc. Most often given to women but can be useful for men and children. The bottled up anger can make them tremble and unable to sleep. Useful for the after effects of invasive or painful operations, ie. those to sphincters or with lacerations (caesarean section).

Physical

Head:	Headaches following grief.
Eyes:	Painful styes.
Urinary:	Cystitis after intercourse.
Women:	Painfully sensitive genitals. Ill effects of rape. Lacerations to perineum.
Worse For:	Suppressed anger, emotions. Sexual excess.
Compare:	Ignatia, Natrum mur.

STRAMONIUM   DATURA STRAMONIUM

Common Name: Thorn-apple
Made From: Potentised tincture of fresh plant in flower and fruit.

Mental & General

A remedy for a violent reaction to a terrifying situation. Fear affects the person profoundly after seeing a death, violence or life-threatening situation. They become terrified of the dark, must sleep with the light on and may wake with night terrors. They cannot bear to be left alone because of the fear. They are afraid of the fear itself, it is so overwhelming. It is mainly a remedy given to children but may be given to adults who react in this way. The person develops a stammer after fright, or gets convulsions. They may become prone to violent impulses and fits of rage.

Physical

Head:	Headache with vertigo. Meningitis. Convulsions. Sun headache.
Eyes:	Staring expression. Objects look black.
Sleep:	Nightmares. Cannot sleep alone or in the dark.
Fever:	Violent fever that nothing relieves. Delusions.
Worse For:	Fright. After sleep. Shining or glistening objects.
Better For:	Light. Company.
Compare:	Aconite, Belladonna, Opium.

SULPHUR SULPHUR

Common Name: Brimstone
Made From: Potentised trituration of flowers of Sulphur.

Mental & General

Mainly used for skin and digestive problems. The action of Sulphur is to assist the body in throwing disease symptoms out of the system. Useful where healing begins but recovery is incomplete (similar to Silica, but Silica is a chilly remedy and Sulphur is a hot remedy). Other remedies help partially but never seem to get to the heart of the case. Complaints go away temporarily but keep returning. The person who needs Sulphur will usually look scruffy, untidy and dirty and their skin will look unhealthy. They are prone to skin complaints that cause itching and burning. Affected parts become red and sore looking. An important remedy for diarrhoea and dysentery, especially that lingers or keeps returning.

Physical

Stomach: Hungry all the time. Suddenly hungry at 11am. Empty and weak feeling in the stomach. Nausea. Vomiting of undigested food.

Abdomen & Stools: Soreness in liver area or abdomen. Jaundice. Colic. Haemorrhoids that itch, burn and bleed. Diarrhoea is worse in the morning; drives the person out of bed. The smell of diarrhoea is horribly offensive. Dysentery. Diarrhoea alternating with constipation.

Respiration: Difficult, irregular breathing. Must have the windows open; craves air. Shooting or burning pains in chest. Rattling cough. Neglected coughs.

Skin: Looks rough, dry, scaly, unhealthy. Itching skin conditions, worse at night, worse in bed and worse after bathing. Skin breaks out and will not heal. Ulcers.

Fever: Flushes of heat. Profuse sweat. Septic fevers.

Worse For: Heat. Suppressions. Bathing. Over-exertion. 11am. Standing.

Better For: Open air. Sweating.

TARENTULA TARENTULA HISPANIA

Common Name: Tarentula, Spanish Spider
Made From: Potentised tincture of the whole poisonous spider.

Mental & General

A remedy for toxaemia and sepsis. The affected part becomes hard and with atrocious burning and stinging pains. It may become bluish purple or red. The pains may cause twitching or jerking. The remedy helps to evacuate pus rapidly. Consider for: malignant ulcers, boils, gangrene, carbuncles. Cutaneous anthrax. The person becomes rapidly weak and tends to sweat copiously. They may be very restless. There is a violence to the symptoms.

Physical

Respiration: Attacks of suffocation. Gagging cough.
Must have fresh air.
Extremities: Restless. Twitching and contractions.
Sawing bone pains.
Skin: Purplish. Pustular eruptions. Itching and crawling.
Excrutiating burning pains in infections.
Fever: Alternating chill and heat.
Worse For: Touch.
Better For: Sweating. Rubbing. Open air.

VERATRUM ALB   VERATRUM ALBUM

Common Name: White Hellebore
Made From: Potentised tincture of the root before flowering.

Mental & General

A remedy marked by copious evacuations and rapid prostration. Coldness and collapse are rapid. Cold sweat on the forehead. Effects are violent and sudden with vomiting, diarrhoea and collapse. Cholera. Fainting from emotion, or with diarrhoea or haemorrhage. Post operative shock. Symptoms may come on after a fright, disappointment, injured pride or honour.

Physical

Face: Looks deathly pale or bluish.
Stomach: Burning thirst especially for ice cold water.
             Craves cold and sour things.
             Excessive vomiting, violent retching. Vomiting
             and purging. Hunger but eating or drinking causes
             nausea and vomiting.
Abdomen & Stools: Painful retraction of abdomen when vomit-
             ing. Stools watery, green or colourless (rice water).
             Stools in large masses. Strains until exhausted,
             with cold sweat. Diarrhoea from drinking cold
             water on hot days or when heated. Cutting colic.
             Peritonitis. Interssusception.
Extremities: Cramps.
Fever: Icy coldness, on head. Internal heat but externally
             cold. Cold sweats.
Worse For: Exertion. Drinking. Cold drinks. Injured pride.
Compare: Arsenicum, Podophyllum.

APPENDICES

HERBAL REMEDIES FOR FIRST AID

	Arnica	Balm	Calendula	Chamomile	Comfrey	Echinacea	Garlic	Lavender Oil	Marshmallow	Plantain	St Johns Wort	Slippery Elm	Tea Tree Oil	Thyme	Yarrow
Bites & Stings		1	2	1		1	2	1	2	1	1		1	2	2
Bruises	1		2	2	1		2			2		2			2
Burns & Scalds			1	1	1	1		1	1	2	1	2	1		
Colds		2		1		1	1	2		1			1	1	1
Conjunctivitis			2	1	2				2	2					
Earache		2		1		1	1	1					2	2	2
Fever		1	2	1		2		1		1			1	1	1
Flu				2		1	1	2		1			1	2	1
Fractures	1				1				2		2				
Nose Bleed			2												1
Shock		1		1				1			2	2	2		
Sprains & Strains	1		2	1			1			2	2		1	2	
Sore Throat		2		2		1	2	1	2			1	2	1	2
Sunburn			2	1	1	1		1	1	1	1	2	2		
Travel Sickness		2		1				1						2	
Wounds			1	2	1	1	1	1	2	1	1	2	1	1	1

1= Most indicated, 2= Appropriate

HOMŒOPATHY FOR ACUTE ILLNESSES

COLIC

Chamomilla	Infants especially. Great irritability and restlessness. May have diarrhoea.
Colocynth	Violent griping pains. Patient bends double or uses pressure to relieve pain. Worse anger.
Mag phos	Cramping, spasmodic pains. Pain better warmth or rubbing.
Nux vomica	Worse after spicy food. Colic with constipation.

CYSTITIS

Apis	Last few drops when urinating are burning and stinging.
Cantharis	Severe stabbing, cutting pains during and after urination. Constant desire to urinate.
Nux vomica	Urge to urinate but cannot pass water. Spasmodic pains.
Staphysagria	Symptoms develop after sexual intercourse or following surgery to genito-urinary tract.

DIARRHOEA
This is best divided into several categories:

Food poisoning Short lasting/watery

Arsenicum	Burning watery diarrhoea. Prostration and restlessness.
China	Profuse diarrhoea. Causes exhaustion.
Colocynth	Diarrhoea with violent griping pains.
Podophyllum	Painless gushing diarrhoea follows gurgling in abdomen. Worse early morning.

Giardiasis — Persistent/watery

Arsenicum	Burning pains passing stool. Prostration and anxiety.
China	Flatulence. Foul stools. Diarrhoea causes depletion and exhaustion.
Pulsatilla	Pale, slimy stools. Pressure sensation in abdomen.
Sulphur	Foul smelling diarrhoea. Worse early morning. Other remedies fail to work.

Dysentery — Bloody diarrhoea

Arsenicum	Burning pains passing stool. Prostration and restlessness.
Baptisia	Severe, prolonged cases. Patient becomes confused, drowsy and collapse threatens.
Colocynth	Violent griping pains with diarrhoea. Rectal spasm.
Ipecac	Excessive blood in stool. Feels feverish. Nausea.
Mercurius	Bloody extremely offensive stools. Continuous urging to stool. Worse night.
Sulphur	Persistent cases. Diarrhoea worse in morning. Other remedies fail to work.

Cholera

Arsenicum	Milder cases and early stages. Burning pains. Prostration and restlessness.
Camphor	Rice water stools. Coldness, blueness and collapse.
Carbo veg	Severe cholera and late stages. Collapse. Patient shocked and almost pulseless.
Veratrum alb	Patient is extremely cold. Cold sweat. Rice water stools.

EARACHE

Aconite	Develops suddenly. Worse after exposure to cold, dry wind.
Belladonna	Throbbing pain in ear. Fever.
Chamomilla	Develops during teething. Child irritable and demanding.
Hepar sulph	Very painful, cannot bear to be touched. Pain worse swallowing.
Pulsatilla	Child becomes tearful and clingy. May be discharge from ear. Develops following a cold.
Silica	Severe or prolonged cases. Mastoiditis threatens. Perforated eardrum.

FEVERS

Aconite	Sudden onset. Patient anxious and fearful. Starts after exposure to cold wind or fright.
Arsenicum	Fever alternates with chill. Restless, anxious patient. Marked weakness.
Baptisia	Prolonged or septic fevers. Prostration. Heaviness and aching of muscles. Dull and confused.
Belladonna	Most common remedy for acute fevers. Burning heat. Delirium. Throbbing headache.
Crotalus horridus	Septic fevers with malignancy. Yellow fever. Black water fever.
Pulsatilla	Fevers in children. Child craves attention. Thirstless.

FLU

Arsenicum	Feverishness alternates with chills. Restless, weak and exhausted.Burning pains.
Eupatorium	Bones ache as though broken. Violent shaking chill.
Gelsemium	Most common remedy. Muscles ache. Chills and fever. Heavy headache.

MALARIA

Arsenicum	Most common remedy. Fever alternating with chills. Prostration.
China	Marked periodicity of attacks. Drenching, debilitating sweats. Symptoms return months later.
Eupatorium	Severe bone pains. Coldness and shivering predominate. Heavy headache.
Natrum mur	Hammering headache. Hives. Homœopathic or orthodox remedies fail to work.
Pulsatilla	Rapidly changing symptoms. Erratic temperature. Diarrhoea.

SEPTIC CONDITIONS

Arsenicum	Burning pains. Restlessness. Part becomes black.
Baptisia	Septicaemia. Low fever. Sore, heavy, aching muscles. Drowsiness, confusion and prostration.
Belladonna	Infections developing with redness, heat and throbbing pains. High temperature, delerium.

Crotalus horridus	Putrid and malignant conditions. Gangrene. Profound nervous shock.
Hepar sulph	Suppurating wounds. Copious pus. Abscess. Touchy mentally and physically.
Hypericum	Bites or stings become infected. Very painful wounds. Prophylactic for tetanus.
Lachesis	Part becomes bluish, mottled or livid. Ulcers. Tissue or blood decomposes. Flushes of heat.
Pyrogen	Rapidly fluctuating temperature. Septicaemia. Foul discharge. Chronic complaints following sepsis.
Silica	Stubborn or chronic infections. Slow development of abscesses etc. Tissue becomes hard or lumpy.
Tarentula	Part becomes hard and excrutiatingly painful. Copious pus.

SORE THROATS

Aconite	Early stages. Fears a cold is developing.
Belladonna	Throat red, sore and swollen. Fever. Threatening tonsillitis.
Ferrum phos	Throat sore and inflamed. Hoarseness.
Hepar sulph	Very painful sore throat. Scraping sensation. Swollen glands. Patient chilly and irritable.
Mercurius	Sore, raw throat with swollen glands. Painful swallowing. Horribly offensive breath.

VOMITING

Arsenicum	Vomiting and purging. Food poisoning. Burning pains.
Nux vomica	Feels better after vomiting then nausea builds up again. Irritability.
Phosphorus	Vomiting worse a few moments after any food or drink. Desires cold drinks.
Pulsatilla	Vomits food eaten much earlier. Worse after rich or fatty food. Thirstless.

SURVIVAL KIT

This is the minimum list of things recommended to have to hand.

HOMŒOPATHIC REMEDIES

Most homœopathic pharmacies supply First Aid Kits containing the most useful remedies. One of the best is the "Basics" Kit supplied by Helios Pharmacy. If you want to put a kit together yourself, it should contain at least the following remedies in 30c potency:

Aconite, Arnica, Arsenicum, Belladonna, Gelsemium, Hypericum, Ledum, Nux vomica, Rhus tox

ESSENTIAL OILS

Citronella: A mosquito repellant that can be diluted and applied to the skin or burnt in a room.
Lavender: Antiseptic and anti-inflammatory. Pour neat onto minor burns and scalds. Hold near the nose and inhale for shock and faintness. Add a few drops to the bath for stress or insomnia.

TINCTURES

Echinacea: Antimicrobial and immunostimulant. Take internally and use externally for any infections: viral or bacterial.
Hypericum and Calendula: An antiseptic and healing lotion. Dab on neat for small cuts, bites, spots, etc. To clean wounds dilute a few drops in a little cool, boiled water and gently bathe the area.

OINTMENTS

Arnica: Bruises. Sprains and strains.
Hypericum and Calendula: A general purpose antiseptic and healing cream. Apply to abrasions, cuts, spots, minor burns, insect bites, etc.

SUNDRIES

Scissors, Sterile Dressings, Safety Pins, Plasters

CONTACTS AND SUPPLIERS

CONTACTS
To find a professional practitioner contact one of the organisations listed below.

HOMŒOPATHY

UK
Society of Homeopaths
2 Artizan Road
Northampton NN1 4HU
Tel: 01604 21400
www.homeopathy-soh.org

The UK Homœopathic Medical Association
6 Livingstone Road
Gravesend
Kent DA12 5DZ
Tel: 01474 560336
www.the-hma.org

Frontline Homeopathy
Ashdale Park House
Donyatt, Illminster
Somerset TA19 ORN
Tel: 01460 52113
www.frontlinehomeopathy.org
Charity that provides homœopathy in communities disadvantaged by social, economic and political circumstances.

USA
National Centre for Homeopathy
www.homeopathic.org

AROMATHERAPY

UK
Aromatherapy Organisations Council
PO Box 355
Croydon CR9 2QP
Tel: 020 8251 7912
www.aocuk.net

USA
The National Association for Holistic Aromatherapy (NAHA)
2000 2nd Avenue, Suite 206
Seattle, WA 98121
Tel: 206-256-0741
www.NAHA.org

HERBALISM

UK
National Institute of Medical Herbalists
56 Longbrook Street
Exeter
Devon EX4 6AH
Tel: 01392 426022
www.nimh.org.uk

USA
The American Association of Naturopathic Physicians
8201 Greensboro Drive, Suite 300
McLean, VA 22102
Tel: 703 610-9037
www.naturopathic.org

SUPPLIERS

UK
Neal's Yard Remedies
15 Neal's Yard
Covent Garden
London WC2H 9DP
Tel: 020 7379 7222
Mail Order: 0161 831 7875
www.nealsyardremedies.com
Suppliers of medicinal herbs and tinctures, essential oils, flower essences, books, etc. through regional shops, mail order and website.

Homœopathic Remedies
Health food shops and pharmacies sell the most popular homœopathic remedies. For more specialised remedies contact one of the
homœopathic pharmacies listed below.

Helios Homœopathic Pharmacy
97 Camden Road
Tunbridge Wells
Kent TN1 2QR
Tel: 01892 536393
www.helios.co.uk
Mail order service available.

Ainsworths Homœopathic Pharmacy
36 New Cavendish Street
London W1M 7LH
Tel: 020 7935 5330
www.ainsworths.com
Mail order service available.

USA
A list of suppliers of herbal remedies is available on
www.herbnet.com

Homeopathic Educational Services
2124 Kittredge St
Berkeley, CA 94704
Tel: (800)359-9051/(510)649-1955
www.homeopathic.com
Homœopathic remedies and books. Mail order service available.

Hahnemann Labs Inc
1940 Fourth Street
San Rafael, CA 94901
Tel: (888)427-6422
www.hahnemannlabs.com
Homœopathic remedies. Mail order service available.

SUGGESTED READING

Barker, J., The Medicinal Flora (London: Winter Press, 2001)

Bartram, T., Encyclopedia of Herbal Medicine (England: Grace, 1995)

Castro, M., The Complete Homœopathy Handbook (London: Macmillan, 1990)

Curtis, S., Homœopathic Alternatives to Immunisation (London: Winter Press, 1994)

Curtis, S., Essential Oils (London: Haldane Mason, 1996)

Davidson, J., Radiation (England: C.W.Daniel, 1986)

Hili, P., Antimicrobial Properties of Essential Oils (London: Winter Press, 2001)

Phatak, S., Materia Medica of Homœopathic Medicines (Delhi: IBPS, 1977)

Shepherd, D., Homœopathy in Epidemic Diseases (Saffron Walden: C.W. Daniel, 1967)

Shepherd, D., Homœopathy for the First Aider (England: C.W.Daniel)

Werner, D., Where There is no Doctor (London: Macmillan 1992)

Wiseman, J., The SAS Survival Handbook (London: Collins Harvill, 1986)

INDEX

Shock 6, 7, 8, 9, 11, 47, 52, 57,
    59, 72, 79, 80, 92
Shooting 7
Siberian ginseng 20
Silica 88, 90
Sinusitis 55, 75
Slippery elm 11, 14, 28, 29, 53
Smallpox 3, 11, 14, 15, 37, 58, 85
Sore throat 45, 55, 58, 61, 65,
    69, 71, 76
Spine 71
Splinters 88
Sprains 29, 30, 41, 44, 62, 75, 85
Staphysagria 7, 88
Stramonium 7, 89
Streptococcus 55
Stress 7, 42, 47, 52, 80
Styes 46, 58, 83, 89
Suicidal 75, 77
Sulphur 90
Sunstroke 61, 69, 89
Symphytum – see Comfrey

Tarentula 14, 91
Tea tree 23, 32, 54
Teeth 49, 51, 66, 75
Teething 66
Terror 11, 89
Terrorism 1, 10, 13, 15
Tetanus 8, 39, 63, 71, 75
Thrush 47, 49, 51, 54, 76
Thyroid 18, 19
Thyme 23, 32, 55
Tinctures 27, 33
Tinnitus 67
Tonsillitis 45, 55, 58, 61, 71, 74, 76
Typhoid 70, 84, 85

Ulcers 29, 44, 45, 49, 50, 51, 53,
    60, 64, 65, 70, 74, 75, 81, 84,
    86, 90, 91
Urticaria 56, 60, 77, 85
Unconscious 59, 63, 79

Vaccines 14, 15, 84
Vaccinia 14
Variolinum 15, 37
Vaseline 9, 31
Veratrum alb 92
Vertigo 62, 70, 72, 75, 77, 80, 89
Vets 38
Victims 7, 88
Vinegar 29
Violent 61, 70, 75, 78, 89
Viruses 45, 46, 54
Vitamin C 18
Vitamin E 18
Vomiting 16, 57, 58, 60, 62, 64,
    68, 69, 73, 78, 81, 82, 84, 90,
    92

Weepy 83
Whooping cough 2, 38, 46, 55,
    58, 64, 73
Wild crafting 24
Wild indigo 13
Worms 46, 55
Worry 62
Wounds 7, 8, 9, 32, 44, 45, 46, 47,
    49, 51, 53, 54, 56, 61, 71, 75

X-ray 16, 37, 84

Yarrow 56
Yersinia pestis 13, 14
Yellow fever 64, 69, 84